The Polyvagal Theory

The Complete Self-Help Guide to Manage Emotional Stress, Trauma, Phobias, Anxiety and Depression

© Copyright 2020 by LAYNE KELLY

All rights reserved

This document is geared towards providing exact and reliable information with regard to the topic and issue covered. The publication is sold with the idea that the publisher is not required to render accounting, officially permitted or otherwise qualified services. If advice is necessary, legal, or professional, a practiced individual in the profession should be ordered. From a Declaration of Principles which was accepted and approved equally by a Committee of the American Bar Association and a Committee of Publishers and Associations.

In no way is it legal to reproduce, duplicate, or transmit any part of this document in either electronic means or in printed format. Recording of this publication is strictly prohibited and any storage of this document is not allowed unless with written permission from the publisher. All rights reserved.

The information provided herein is stated to be truthful and consistent, in that any liability, in terms of inattention or otherwise, by any usage or abuse of any policies, processes, or directions contained within is the solitary and utter responsibility of the recipient reader. Under no circumstances will any legal responsibility or blame be held against the publisher for any reparation, damages, or monetary loss due to the information herein, either directly or indirectly.

Respective authors own all copyrights not held by the publisher.

The information herein is offered for informational purposes solely and is universal as so. The presentation of the information is without a contract or any type of guarantee assurance.

The trademarks that are used are without any consent, and the publication of the trademark is without permission or backing by the trademark owner. All trademarks and brands within this book are for clarifying purposes only and are owned by the owners themselves, not affiliated with this document

TABLE OF CONTENTS

INTRODUCTION 1

CHAPTER ONE: POLYVAGAL THEORY IN PRACTICE 5

Our three-section sensory system 6

Injury's impact on sensory system reaction 9

Explicit parts of ventral vagal nerve working 12

Polyvagal theory 14

CHAPTER TWO: POLYVAGAL THEORY AND HOW IT RELATES TO SOCIAL CUES 18

The Body's Surveillance System 19

Perusing Danger Cues 21

The Vagus Nerve 22

Three Developmental Stages of Response 25

CHAPTER THREE: POLYVAGAL THEORY SIMPLIFIED 32

Association Mode 35

Freeze, Flight, Fight, or Puff Up 37

How injury influences the sensory system 41

CHAPTER FOUR: CHILDREN, EMOTIONAL REGULATION, AND POLYVAGAL THEORY 55

Being a sentiments analyst 56

Polyvagal theory and kids 57

Tools for passionate guideline 61

Bringing up Resilient Children 66

Strength is for Parents Too 68

CHAPTER FIVE: POLYVAGAL THEORY AND ANXIETY 71

Why Your Personal Narrative Adds To The Problem 76

An Every Day Breathing Technique You Can Use Anywhere 80

CHAPTER SIX: POLYVAGAL THEORY AND PTSD 82

The Sensory System: A Basic Model 82

Bioconductal Defenses 85

The Vagal Brake 86

The Social Sensory System 87

Suggestions for Healing PTSD 91

Settling Complex PTSD and Dissociation 96

CHAPTER SEVEN: THE VAGAL PARADOX 100

Consistency with Jacksonian Dissolution 106

Different supporters of neuroception 114

CHAPTER EIGHT: DORSAL VAGAL, FREEZE, AND POLYVAGAL SOLUTIONS 116

The Role of the Dorsal Vagal and Pain 118

Methodologies to Shift out of Maladaptive Defense States 121

The Importance of Breathing and Movement 127

The HPA (Hypothalamic Pituitary Adrenal Axis) 133

Dread and Depression, Polyvagal Science, and Pain 137

The Dorsal Vagal Shutdown 153

CHAPTER NINE: CLINICAL APPLICATIONS OF THE POLYVAGAL THEORY 162

Reframe Your Thinking Around Autism 165

CHAPTER TEN: YOGA TREATMENT AND THE POLYVAGAL THEORY 167

Vagal Activity, Interoception, Regulation, and Resilience 178

Polyvagal Theory & Mind-Body Therapies for Regulation & Resilience 181

SUMMARY 185

CONCLUSION 194

INTRODUCTION

The polyvagal theory portrays an autonomic sensory system that is impacted by the focal sensory system, touchy to afferent impacts, described by a versatile reactivity reliant on the phylogeny of the neural circuits, and intelligent with source cores in the brainstem managing the striated muscles of the face and head.

The theory is reliant on collected information portraying the phylogenetic advances in the vertebrate autonomic sensory system.

Its particular spotlight is on the phylogenetic move among reptiles and warm-blooded animals that brought about explicit changes to the vagal pathways directing the heart. As the source cores of the essential vagal efferent pathways managing the heart moved from the dorsal engine core of the vagus in reptiles to the core ambiguous in warm-blooded creatures, a face-heart association developed with rising properties of a social commitment framework that would empower social communications to control instinctive state.

Focal sensory system guideline of instinctive organs is the focal point of a few noteworthy distributions that have molded the surface of physiological request. For instance, in 1872, Darwin recognized the dynamic neural connection between the heart and the mind:

. . .at the point when the heart is influenced it responds on the mind; and the condition of the brain again responds through the pneumo-gastric [vagus] nerve on the heart; so that under any fervor there will be a lot of common activity and response between these, the two most significant organs of the body.

In spite of the fact that Darwin recognized the bidirectional correspondence between the viscera and the brain, resulting in a formal portrayal of the autonomic sensory system limited the significance of focal administrative structures and afferents. Following Langley, clinical and physiological research would, in general, spotlight on the fringe engine nerves of the autonomic anxious system, with a theoretical accentuation on the matched threat among thoughtful and parasympathetic efferent pathways on the objective instinctive organs. This center limited enthusiasm for both afferent pathways and the brainstem regions that manage explicit efferent pathways.

The early conceptualization of the vagus concentrated on an undifferentiated efferent pathway that was accepted to balance "tone" simultaneously to a few objective organs. In this way, brainstem zones controlling the supradiaphragmatic (e.g., myelinated vagal pathways beginning in the core ambiguous and ending fundamentally over the stomach) were not practically recognized from those directing the subdiaphragmatic (e.g., unmyelinated vagal pathways starting in the dorsal engine core of the vagus and ending principally underneath the stomach). Without this differentiation, research and theory concentrated on the combined hostility between the parasympathetic and thoughtful innervation to the target organs. The outcome of accentuation on matched opposition was an acknowledgment in physiology and medication of worldwide builds, for example, autonomic equalization, thoughtful tone, and vagal tone.

Over 50 years back, Hess recommended that the autonomic sensory system was not exclusively vegetative and programmed but rather was rather a coordinated framework with both fringe and focal neurons. By underlining the focal components that intervene in the dynamic guideline of fringe organs, Hess foresaw the requirement for advances to ceaselessly screen fringe and focal neural circuits engaged with the guideline of instinctive capacity.

CHAPTER ONE: POLYVAGAL THEORY IN PRACTICE

Picturing brain chemistry can be something like envisioning a tropical storm. Although we can envision a terrible climate, it is hard to envision changing that climate. However, Stephen Porges' polyvagal theory gives advocates a valuable image of the sensory system that can direct us in our endeavors to support customers.

Porges' polyvagal theory created out of his examinations with the vagus nerve. The vagus nerve serves the parasympathetic sensory system, which is the quieting part of our sensory system mechanics. The parasympathetic piece of the autonomic sensory system adjusts the thoughtful dynamic part, yet is considerably more nuanced ways than we comprehended before polyvagal theory.

Our three-section sensory system

Before polyvagal theory, our sensory system was imagined as a two-section opposing framework, with more initiation flagging not so much quieting but rather more quieting flagging less enactment. The polyvagal theory distinguishes the third sort of sensory system reaction that is called the social commitment framework, a lively blend of actuation and quieting that works out of one of a kind nerve impact.

The social commitment framework encourages us to explore connections. Helping our customers move into the utilization of their social commitment framework permits them to turn out to be progressively adaptable in their adapting styles.

The two different pieces of our sensory system capacity to assist us with overseeing dangerous circumstances, most advisors are now acquainted with the two guard instruments activated by these two pieces of the sensory system: thoughtful battle or-flight and parasympathetic shutdown, now and again called freeze-or-black out. Utilization of our social commitment framework, then again, requires a feeling of wellbeing.

Polyvagal theory causes us to comprehend that the two parts of the vagus nerve quiet the body, yet they do as such in various manners. Shutdown, or freeze-or-black out, happens through the dorsal part of the vagus nerve. This response can feel like the exhausted muscles and discombobulation of an awful influenza. At the point when the dorsal vagal nerve closes down the body, it can move us into stability or separation. Notwithstanding influencing the heart and lungs, the dorsal branch influences the body working underneath the stomach and is associated with stomach related problems.

The central part of the vagal nerve influences the body working over the stomach. This is the branch that serves the social commitment framework. The ventral vagal nerve hoses the body's consistently dynamic state. Picture controlling a pony as you ride it back to the stable. You would keep on pulling back on and discharge the reins in nuanced approaches to guarantee that the pony keeps up a proper speed. In like manner, the ventral vagal nerve permits initiation in a nuanced way, in this way offering an unexpected quality in comparison to thoughtful enactment.

Ventral vagal discharge into movement takes milliseconds, while thoughtful actuation takes seconds and includes different synthetic responses that are much the same as losing the pony's reins. What's more, when the battle or-flight compound responses have started, it can take our bodies 10–20 minutes to come back to our pre-battle/pre-flight state. Ventral vagal discharge into movement doesn't include these sorts of synthetic responses. Subsequently, we can make snappier alterations among initiation and quieting, like what we can do when we utilize the reins to control the pony.

In the event that you go to a canine park, you will see certain pooches that are apprehensive. They display battle or-flight practices. Different mutts will flag a desire to play. This flagging frequently takes the structure that we people seized for the descending confronting hound present in yoga. At the point when a canine gives this sign, it signals a degree of excitement that can be extraordinary. Be that as it may, this perky vitality has an altogether different soul than the force of battle or-flight practices. This energetic soul portrays the social commitment framework. At the point when we experience our condition as protected, we work from our social commitment framework.

Injury's impact on sensory system reaction

On the off chance that we have uncertain injury from quite a while ago, we may live in the form of ceaseless battle or-flight. We might have the option to channel this battle or-flight uneasiness into exercises, for example, cleaning the house, raking the forgets about or working at the rec center, yet these exercises will have an unexpected vibe in comparison to they would on the off chance that they were finished with social commitment science (think "Whistle While You Work").

For some injury survivors, no movement effectively channels their battle or-flight sensations. Therefore, they feel caught and their bodies shut down. These customers may live in a rendition of a never-ending shutdown.

Levine has considered the shutdown reaction through creature perceptions and bodywork with customers. He clarifies that rising up out of shutdown requires a shiver or shake to release suspended battle or-flight vitality. In a perilous circumstance, on the off chance that we have shut down and an open door for dynamic endurance introduces itself, we can wake ourselves up. As advisors, we may perceive this move from shutdown to battle or-trip in a customer's move from wretchedness into tension.

However, how might we help our customers move into their social commitment science? In the event that customers live in an increasingly dissociative, discouraged, shutdown way, we should assist them with moving briefly into battle or-flight. As customers experience battle or-flight power, we should then assist them with finding a feeling of security. At the point when they can detect that they are protected, they can move into their social commitment framework.

The body-mindfulness procedures that are a piece of cognitive conduct treatment (CBT) and dialectical conduct treatment (DBT) can assist customers with moving out of dissociative, shutdown reactions by urging them to turn out to be progressively typified. At the point when customers are increasingly present in their bodies and better ready to take care of transient solid strain, they can wake up from a shutdown reaction. As customers actuate out of shutdown and move toward battle or-flight sensations, the idea rebuilding methods that are additionally part of CBT and DBT can instruct customers to assess their security all the more precisely. Intelligent listening systems can assist customers with feeling an association with their advocates. This causes it feasible for these customers to feel sufficiently safe to move into social commitment science.

Explicit parts of ventral vagal nerve working

Porges picked the name social commitment framework on the grounds that the ventral vagal nerve influences the center ear, which sift through foundation clamors to make it simpler to hear the human voice. It additionally influences facial muscles and therefore the capacity to make informative outward appearances. At long last, it influences the larynx and hence vocal tone and vocal designing, helping people make sounds that calm each other.

Customers with poor social commitment framework working may have inward ear challenges that make it difficult for them to get relieving from others' voices. As guides, we can be aware of our vocal examples and outward appearances and inquisitive about the impacts those parts of our correspondence have on our customers.

In view of his comprehension of the impacts of the vagus nerve, Porges takes note of that broadening breathes out longer than breathes in for a while actuates the parasympathetic sensory system. Porges that was a clarinet player in his childhood recalls the impact of the breath designs required to play that instrument.

As a moving advisor, I am mindful that expanding breathes out helps customers who are stuck in types of battle or-flight reaction to move into a feeling of wellbeing. For customers stuck in some type of shutdown, I have discovered that cognizant breath-work can mix the battle or flight reaction. At the point when this happens, the battle or-flight vitality should be released through development for customers to discover a feeling of wellbeing. For example, these customers may need to run set up or punch a cushion. The chain of command of resistance framework working clarifies these remedial procedures.

Respiratory sinus arrhythmia is a decent file of ventral vagal working. This implies we presently have strategies to examine the viability of body treatments and expressive expressions treatments.

Polyvagal theory

What follows is a case of how I utilized polyvagal theory with a customer who experienced a clinical injury during her introduction to the world.

The customer, whom I have seen for quite a while, portrayed inclination drowsy and recognized experiencing issues finding a workable pace on this day. Her therapist had recommended her a medicine as a method for treating uneasiness mixed by the introduction of her girl's first youngster. The customer and I had recently standardized her uneasiness as an injury reaction.

During the prior year's coming to see me, this customer had endeavored suicide, which brought about clinical techniques that add to her injury. Through our work, she has come to comprehend that the fits of anxiety she has when in contained circumstances are additionally injury reactions. She has lived quite a bit of her life in interminable battle or-flight reaction mode.

On this day, she was alleviated to be less enthusiastic, yet she dreaded the tiredness that went with medicine's assistance in quieting her battle or-flight sensations. I considered this to be of the tiredness as a dread of a dorsal vagal shutdown. We examined the likelihood that this tiredness could permit her another sort of initiation. I inquired as to whether she might want to do some expressive craftsmanship that would permit delicate, expressive development. She shivered, naming her inclination for things that were less abstract.

We discussed the presence of a sort of aliveness that, despite everything, has a sense of security. We discussed the chance of existing in an energetic spot where there is no good and bad, just inclination. We recognized that since her introduction to the world, she and her folks had expected that her wellbeing would flop once more. This condition, wherein she had grown up, had bolstered sensory system working intended forever undermining circumstances. With medicines quieting her battle or-flight initiation, I recommended that maybe she could investigate some quieter, increasingly fun-loving sorts of emotional encounters.

"It feels like you are attempting to make an alternate me," she reacted. I recognized that it might seem as though I were suspecting she could be somebody she wasn't. Yet, I clarified that what I was really proposing was simply the likelihood that she could be in an alternate manner.

The customer revealed to me she had another book on grand-parenting that contained a part in the play. She said she would think about understanding it. Simultaneously, she said that she probably wouldn't have the option to endure the medicine and might need to get off of it. In any case, the possibility of this unique, increasingly lively method for being has been acquainted with her and, for a minute or two, experienced.

Getting the picture

As instructors equipped with a polyvagal theory, we can picture resistance component chain of command. We can perceive shifts from battle or-trip to close down when customers feel caught. We can likewise perceive the development from shutdown into battle or-flight that offers a potential move into social commitment science if and when the customer can increase a feeling of wellbeing.

Before the polyvagal theory, most instructors could likely perceive battle or-flight and shutdown practices. They could presumably detect contrast between barrier reactions intended forever, compromising circumstances and reactions that are called the social commitment framework. The polyvagal theory extends that mindfulness with the information that fun-loving excitement and therapeutic give up have an interesting sensory system impact.

Most advocates acknowledge brain chemistry; however, they may think that it's hard to picture how to utilize the data. On account of the polyvagal theory's explanation of the job of the central part of the vagus nerve, we presently have a guide to direct us.

CHAPTER TWO: POLYVAGAL THEORY AND HOW IT RELATES TO SOCIAL CUES

Have you at any point been in a circumstance where you feel unsure or in harm's way however not so much sure why? You may glance around and see that nobody else is by all accounts irritated, yet something despite everything feels off to you?

You may not understand it; however, you are strolling around on the planet every day, perusing a great many meaningful gestures in your condition. In our collaboration with others, we get outward appearances, manners of speaking, substantial development, and the sky is the limit from there. We are continually bustling watching and communicating with the world and others as a feature of the human experience.

As we have these communications with others, our feeling of self is being molded. We find out about ourselves and about others, who we can trust, and who feels hazardous to us. Our bodies are preparing this kind of data continually through these associations with the world.

The Body's Surveillance System

Our sensory system is an unpredictable structure that accumulates data from all over our body and facilitates movement. There are two fundamental pieces of the sensory system: the focal sensory system and the fringe sensory system.

Focal Sensory System

The focal sensory system comprises of two structures:

- Brain. This is the structure made out of billions of interconnected neurons or nerve cells contained in the skull and capacities as the planning place for practically the entirety of our body's capacities. It is the seat of our acumen.

- Spinal line. This is a packaged system of nerve filaments, interfacing most pieces of our body to our brain.

Fringe Sensory System

The fringe sensory system comprises the entirety of the nerves outside of our mind and spinal line. It tends to be ordered into two particular frameworks:

- Somatic sensory system (willful). This framework permits our muscles and brains to speak with one another. The physical framework enables our mind and spinal rope to impart signs to our muscles to assist them with moving, just as sends data from the body back to the brain and spinal rope.
- Autonomic sensory system (automatic). This is the framework that controls the organs and interior organs, for example, the heart, lungs, and stomach related framework. These are, basically, the things that run our body without us having to purposefully consider them. For

instance, we can inhale without contemplating taking a breath each time.

Perusing Danger Cues

Our autonomic sensory system (the automatic framework that assists with controlling things like our breathing, pulse, assimilation, and salivation) is unpredictable and constantly occupied. Notwithstanding running these significant capacities in our bodies, for example, helping us inhale, helping our heart siphon, and helping us digest nourishment, our autonomic sensory system is likewise helping us to check, decipher, and react to risk prompts.

There are two separate frameworks grinding away inside the autonomic sensory system that is helping us to peruse and react to risk signals:

- Sympathetic sensory system. This framework is associated with stimulating our bodies to react by activating us to move when in risky circumstances. Many allude to this framework as provoking our "battle or flight" responses to threat signs in our condition. It is likewise liable for enacting our adrenal organs to discharge epinephrine into our circulation system, also called an adrenaline surge. At the point when we see a snake, our thoughtful sensory system will peruse the sign of the potential risk and brief our body to react, likely including a fast adrenaline surge and us promptly moving endlessly from the snake.

- Parasympathetic sensory system. This framework is associated with quieting our bodies, saving vitality as it does things like moderate our pulse, manage our assimilation and lower our circulatory strain. Some allude to this framework as the "rest and summary" framework. As we read that a prompt isn't risky, our body starts to quiet with the assistance of our parasympathetic sensory system.

The Vagus Nerve

There is one nerve, specifically, that is important to The Polyvagal Theory: The vagus nerve.

The vagus nerve is the tenth cranial nerve, a long and meandering nerve that starts at the medulla oblongata. This piece of the brain, the medulla oblongata, is situated in the lower some portion of the mind, sitting simply above where the brain interfaces with our spinal rope.

There are different sides to this vagus nerve, the dorsal (back) and the ventral (front). From that point, the different sides of the vagus nerve run down all through our body, considered to have the most extensive dispersion of the considerable number of nerves inside the human body.

Filtering our Environment

From the time we are conceived, we are instinctively checking our condition for prompts of security and threat.

A child reacts to the sheltered sentiments of closeness with their parent or guardian. In like manner, an infant will react to signals that are seen as unnerving or risky, similar to a more odd, an alarming clamor, or an absence of reaction from their guardian. We filter for signs of wellbeing and peril our whole lives.

Perception

The polyvagal theory depicts the procedure where our neural circuits are perusing prompts of threat in our condition as neuroception. Through this procedure of neuroception, we are encountering the world in a manner by which we are automatically examining circumstances and individuals to decide whether they are sheltered or perilous.

As a component of our autonomic sensory system, this procedure is going on without us in any event, staying alert that it is going on. Similarly, as we can inhale without having to purposefully instruct ourselves to calmly inhale; we can check our condition for prompts without guiding ourselves to do as such. The vagus nerve is specifically noteworthy during this procedure of neuroception.

During the time spent neuroception, the two sides of our vagus nerve can be invigorated. Each side (ventral and dorsal) has been found to react in particular manners as we sweep and procedure data from our condition and social co-operations.

The ventral (front) side of the vagus nerve reacts to prompts of wellbeing in our condition and collaborations. It bolsters sentiments of physical security and being securely sincerely associated with others in our social condition.

The dorsal (posterior of the vagus nerve reacts to signals of peril, it pulls us away from the association, out of mindfulness, and into a condition of self-assurance. In minutes when we may encounter a sign of extraordinary risk, we can close down and feel solidified, a sign that our dorsal vagal nerve has dominated.

Three Developmental Stages of Response

The polyvagal theory portrays three transformative stages engaged with the advancement of our autonomic sensory system. Instead of just proposing that there is a harmony between our thoughtful and parasympathetic sensory system, The theory describe that there is really a chain of command of reactions incorporated with our autonomic sensory system.

- Immobilization. Portrayed as the most seasoned pathway, this includes an immobilization reaction. As you would recollect the dorsal (posterior of the vagus nerve react to signs of extraordinary risk, this implies we would react to our dread by getting solidified, numb, and closing down. As though our parasympathetic sensory system is kicking into overdrive, our reaction really brings about us freezing, as opposed to just backing off.
- Mobilization. Inside this reaction, we are taken advantage of our thoughtful sensory system which, as you may recall, is the framework that causes us to activate notwithstanding a risk signal. We get a move on our adrenaline race to escape from peril or to fend off our risk. The polyvagal theory proposes that this pathway was besides creating in the transformative pecking order.

- Social commitment. The most current expansion to the progression of reactions, this is situated in our ventral (front) side of the vagus nerve. Recollecting that this piece of the vagus nerve reacts to sentiments of wellbeing and association, social commitment permits us to feel secured and is encouraged by that ventral vagus pathway. Right now, you can have a sense of security, quiet, associated, and locked in.

The Response Hierarchy in Daily Life

As we experience life connecting with the world, there are unavoidably those minutes when we will have a sense of security and others or in which we will feel inconvenience or threat. The polyvagal theory proposes that this space is liquid for us and we can move all through these better places inside the progressive system of reactions.

We may encounter social commitment in the grasp of a safe cherished one and, around the same time, wind up in preparation as we are stood up to with threat, for example, an out of control hound, a theft, or an extraordinary clash with an associate.

There are times when we may peruse and react to a risk sign and procedure the circumstance such that drives us to feel caught and incapable of escaping the circumstance. In those minutes, our body is reacting to expanded sentiments of threat and trouble, moving into an increasingly basic space of immobilization. Our dorsal vagus nerve is being affected and securing us to a position of freezing, feeling numb and, as certain scientists accept, separation.

The risk signs can turn out to be excessively overpowering in those minutes and we see no reasonable way out. A case of this could be snapshots of sexual or physical maltreatment.

Effect of Trauma

At the point when somebody has encountered an injury, especially in encounters where they were left immobilized, their capacity to examine their condition for peril prompts can get slanted. Obviously, our body will probably help us never experience an unnerving minute like that again, so it will do whatever it needs to do so as to help secure us.

Our social commitment permits us to associate all the more smoothly with others, feeling associated and safe. At the point when our body gets a prompt inside a collaboration that signals we may not be sheltered, it starts to react. For some, this sign may move them into a position of an activation reaction, getting a move on the endeavor to kill the risk or escape from the danger.

For the individuals who have encountered an injury, the sign of a threat prompt can move them straightforwardly from social commitment to immobilization. Astonishingly partner various relational prompts as risky, for example, a slight difference in outward appearance, a specific manner of speaking, or particular sorts of body posing, they can wind up returning to a position of reaction that is recognizable to them with an end goal to get ready and secure themselves.

A reaction of assembly may not be enrolled by the body as an alternative. This can be very confounding for injury survivors, ignorant of how this pecking order of a reaction is affected by their communications with others and the world.

Association and Polyvagal Theory

In spite of the fact that the vagus nerve is known for being generally circulated and associated with an assortment of regions of the body, note that this framework can impact cranial nerves that control social commitment through outward appearance and vocalization. As people who are wired for association, we can see how filtering for peril prompts can happen every now and again in our communications with our loved one or significant strong others in our lives.

We naturally long for sentiments of wellbeing, trust, and solace in our associations with others and rapidly get prompts that reveal to us when we may not be sheltered. As individuals become more secure with and for one another, it very well may be simpler to manufacture sound bonds, share vulnerabilities, and experience closeness with one another.

CHAPTER THREE: POLYVAGAL THEORY SIMPLIFIED

The polyvagal theory clarifies three distinct pieces of our sensory system and their reactions to distressing circumstances. When we comprehend those three sections, we can perceive any reason why and how we respond to high measures of pressure.

On the off chance that polyvagal theory sounds as energizing as watching paint dry, stay, trust me. It's an entrancing clarification of how our body handles enthusiastic pressure, and how we can utilize various treatments to revise the impact of injury.

For what reason is the polyvagal theory significant?

For specialists and pop-brain research aficionado the same, understanding polyvagal theory can help with:

- Understanding injury and PTSD

- Understanding the move of assault and withdrawal seeing someone
- Understanding how extraordinary pressure prompts separation or closing down
- Understanding how to peruse non-verbal communication

We like to think about our feelings as ethereal, complex, and hard to arrange and distinguish.

In all actuality, feelings are reactions to an improvement (inner or outer). Regularly they occur out of our mindfulness, particularly in the event that we are withdrawn or incongruent, with our internal enthusiastic life.

Our base wants to remain alive. This is essential to our body. That is the place the polyvagal theory comes in to play.

The sensory system is continually running out of sight, controlling our body capacities so we can consider different things—like what sort of dessert we'd prefer to request, or how to get that An in medications school. The whole sensory system works a couple with the brain and can assume control over our enthusiastic experience, regardless of whether we don't need it to.

An anecdote about a gazelle...

Creatures are an incredible case of how we handle pressure, since they respond basely, without mindfulness. They do what we would, on the off chance that we weren't so very much restrained.

On the off chance that you have ever viewed a National Geographic Africa extraordinary, you've seen a lioness pursue a gazelle. A gathering of gazelles is brushing, and out of nowhere, one gazes upward, hyper mindful of what's going on around him, the entire gathering notification and focuses.

After a minute, the lioness begins her pursuit. The gazelle she's singled out runs as quickly as possible (thoughtful sensory system) until he is gotten. At the point when he is gotten, he immediately goes limp (parasympathetic sensory system).

The lioness hauls the gazelle back to her offspring, where they start to play with it before they go in for the murder. In the event that the lioness gets occupied, and the gazelle sees a snapshot of chance, he's up and dashing off once more, seeming as though he unexpectedly returned to life (once more into thoughtful sensory system reaction).

At the point when the gazelle was gotten, with teeth around his neck, his shutdown reaction kicked in - he solidified. Whenever he saw the chance to run, his battle or flight kicked in, and he ran.

The polyvagal theory covers those three states—association, battle or flight, or shutdown.

Here's the way they work...

Association Mode

Or...rest and relaxation...or myelinated vagus nerve of the parasympathetic sensory system originating from the core uncertain reaction

During non-unpleasant circumstances, on the off chance that we are sincerely sound, our bodies remain in a social commitment state, or a cheerful, typical, non-go crazy state.

I like to call it "association." By association, I imply that we are fit for "associated" cooperation with another person. We are strolling near, unafraid, making the most of our day, eating with loved ones and our body and feelings feel typical.

It's likewise called ventral vagal reaction since that is the piece of the mind that is initiated during association mode. It resembles a green light for ordinary life.

What does this look like and feel?

- Our resistant framework is sound.
- We feel typical bliss, transparency, harmony, and interest in existence.
- We are resting soundly and eating typically.
- Our face is expressive.
- We sincerely identify with others.
- We all the more effectively comprehend and tune in to other people.
- Our body feels quiet and grounded.

Freeze, Flight, Fight, or Puff Up

...or on the other hand the thoughtful sensory system reaction

The thoughtful sensory system is our prompt response to push that influences almost every organ in the body.

The thoughtful sensory system causes that "battle or flight" state we have all known about. It gives us those prompts with the goal that it can keep us alive.

How does this occur? What does this look like and feel?

- We sense the risk and stick to check the environmental factors for genuine peril.
- We discharge cortisol, epinephrine and norepinephrine to enable us to achieve what we have to - escape or battle our foe.
- Our heartbeat spikes, we sweat, and we feel more prepared.
- We feel restless, apprehensive, or irate.
- There might be flashes of outward appearances of dread and outrage, with the

foundation of all the more a despite everything face. In the event that positive feelings are available, they generally look constrained.

- Our absorption eases back down as blood races to the muscles.
- Our veins tighten to the digestion tracts and expand to the muscles expected to run or battle.
- We might need to flee, or punch somebody, or respond genuinely here and there, or simply puff-up and look frightening.
- Our muscles may feel tense, electric, tight, vibrating, throbbing, trembling, and hard.
- Our hands might be moist.
- Our stomach might be agonizingly tied.
- All our faculties' center.
- Our motions may show guarding of our crucial organs, clench hands gripped or puffing ourselves up to look greater or more grounded.

In battle or flight, at some level, we accept we can at present endure whatever risk we believe is hazardous.

Close Down

...or then again the Unmyelinated Vagus of the Parasympathetic Sensory System originating from the Dorsal Motor Nucleus

What's intriguing about this piece of the parasympathetic sensory system? Its capacity is to keep us solidified as a versatile instrument to assist us with getting by to either battle or flight once more.

At the point when David Livingston was assaulted by a lion, he later revealed, "it caused a kind of vagueness in which there was no feeling of torment nor sentiment of fear, however very aware of every one of that was going on."

At the point when our thoughtful sensory system has kicked into overdrive, we despite everything can't get away and feel looming passing the dorsal vagal parasympathetic sensory system takes control.

It causes freezing or shutdown, as a type of self-safeguarding. (Consider somebody who drops under outrageous pressure.)

What does this look like and feel?

- Emotionally, it feels like separation, deadness, bleary-eyed, misery, disgrace, a feeling of feeling caught, out of the body, disengaged from the world
- Our eyes may watch fixed and scattered
- The dorsal engine core through the unmyelinated vagus nerve diminishes our pulse, circulatory strain, outward appearances, sexual and resistant reaction frameworks
- We might be activated to feel sickened, hurl, crap, precipitously pee
- We may feel low or no torment
- Our lungs (bronchi) contract and we inhale slower
- We may experience issues getting words out or feel choking around our throat

- Our brain has diminished digestion and this causes lost body mindfulness, limp appendages, diminished capacity to think plainly, and diminished capacity to set down account recollections
- Our body stance may fall or twist up in a ball

In shutdown mode, at some level, our sensory system accepts we are in a hazardous circumstance, and it attempts to keep us alive through keeping our body still.

A few people who have had both connection injury and consequent injury can have ceaseless suicidality and separation scenes that last days to months. Research shows that long haul arrangements include:

- Dialectical conduct treatment
- Mentalization-based treatment
- Transference centered treatment

How injury influences the sensory system

As people, we do a similar thing as that gazelle when we see enthusiastic or physical risk. We switch back and forth between quiet touching (parasympathetic - association mode), battle or flight (thoughtful framework battle and flight) or shutdown (parasympathetic-shut down mode).

Our reaction is all in our view of the occasion. Possibly somebody was simply playing a game when they leaped out to unnerve us, yet we swooned. Whatever the explanation, regardless of whether the episode was purposeful or not, our body moved into shutdown mode, we enrolled it as an injury. Our body moved into shutdown mode.

Or on the other hand, perhaps the injury occasion was true, hazardous, and our sensory system reacted suitably to the boosts.

Regardless of what the reason was, our mind accepted what was going on was dangerous enough that it made our body go into battle, flight, or shutdown mode.

On the off chance that somebody has experienced such a horrendous mishap, that their body tips into shutdown reaction, any occasion that helps the individual to remember that dangerous event can trigger them into disengagement or separation once more.

Individuals can even live in a condition of separation or shut down for a considerable length of time or month's one after another.

Veterans regularly experience this during boisterous, abrupt commotions, for example, firecrackers or tempests. A lady who was assaulted may rapidly switch into the hypervigilant or separated reaction in the event that she feels somebody is following her. Somebody who was manhandled may be activated when much someone else begins shouting.

The issue happens when we haven't prepared the first injury so that the first injury is settled.

That is the thing that PTSD (post-awful pressure issue) is—our body's eruption to a little reaction, and either stuck in battle and flight or shut down.

Individuals who experience injury and the shutdown reaction typically feel disgrace around their failure to act, when their body didn't move. They regularly wish they would have battled more during those minutes.

A Vietnam vet may feel they bombed their partners who passed on around them while they stood, solidified in dread. An unfortunate assault casualty may feel the individual in question didn't fend off their attacker since they solidified. A casualty of misuse may feel they quit attempting to get away from their abuser, and that they are frail or fizzled.

Quite a bit of "stress" preparing, which trains individuals to keep on staying in battle and flight mode, intends to keep individuals out of separation during the reality of passing circumstances. Sadly, these practices aren't regular past world-class sports groups or unique powers. The perfect measure of worry, with great recuperation, can lead our sensory systems into more significant levels of adjustment.

Leaving shutdown mode

So how would we move to pull out of shutdown mode?

Something contrary to the dorsal vagal framework is the social commitment framework.

In this way, to put it plainly, what fixes shutdown mode is bringing somebody into sound social commitment, or legitimate connection.

Getting down into the stray pieces of how this functions in our body can assist us with understanding why we feel the manner in which we do truly when your body is in battle, flight, or shut down mode.

At the point when we comprehend why our body responds to the manner in which it does, similar to a series of signs and some fundamental science about the brain, we can see how to switch states. We can start to move out of the battle or flight state, out of the shutdown mode, and go into the social commitment state.

As specialists, regardless of whether we are simply setting up an association with another, on edge patients, or helping them manage their most profound horrendous recollections, realizing how to explore the polyvagal states is significant.

It can likewise be useful in the event that you have recently distinguished yourself in a portion of these side effects. For example, "When I'm with my folks, even as an Adult and they begin battling, I feel dizzy and disengaged."

In the event that you've seen a portion of these things in yourself, ideally through treatment, and in any event, seeing how this works, you can haul yourself out of a disengaged state.

Studies show that a few pieces of the mind shut down during the review of awful accidents, including the verbal focuses and the thinking places of the brain.

This is the reason it's essential to direct treatment, or leaving shutdown mode, in a sheltered, sound way, in a protected, solid condition. This is the reason a positive connection is basic. Else, you risk re-traumatizing the patient.

Since I am a specialist, I will compose this to exhibit how to enable a patient change to out of shutdown mode.

Nonetheless, these tips despite everything apply to the individuals who are simply seeing how shutdown mode functions. Furthermore, it can even assist the individuals who feel shut down to start to realize how to attempt to achieve a sound social commitment mode once more.

- Have a trust-based relationship. Due to the possibility to re-damage, don't address seriously awful mishaps—particularly ones where you think shutdown mode kicked in until the helpful relationship feels profoundly associated.

It's significant as the specialist to permit the patient to communicate things they couldn't communicate to others—despicable sentiments, outrage, sexual reaction, anything that feels startling to impart to other people.

- Find your own quiet place. On the off chance that you can identify with their misery, remain at the time with them, and assist them with feeling associated during their shutdown, you are tossing them a lifesaver. You're helping them leave shutdown, into social commitment.

It's critical to the battle against the inclination to separate, regardless of how abhorrent the topic is. As advisors, we could separate due to the mirror neuron reaction - to reflect our patient's mind, and in light of the fact that when hearing horrendous injury, it's anything but difficult to envision it transpiring.

The human experience is amazing to such an extent that when we reconnect the injury, with another person to help us, it revamps that occasion in our brain, including the sentiment of being bolstered inside the injury memory. We make new neural pathways around the injury, and we can change our body's reaction to it.

- Let the patient lead. Try not to go on a witch chase. On the off chance that the patient brings it up, incline toward the subject. Be that as it may, it is destructive to incite the patient into something that isn't there by posing driving inquiries and attempting to get them to admit. Try not to let your own experience lead you to envision they have additionally experienced something.
- Normalize their reaction. The whole polyvagal theory should make our state "thank you!" to our bodies, regardless of whether that framework is overactive now and again - baseless frenzy - that our body is looking out for us, attempting to keep us alive.

Our body responding in that manner is a similar thing as the gazelle either fleeing or going limp. What's more, gazelles have no clue what feelings are in any case.

Since the patient comprehends that their passionate reaction was versatile, base, and fitting, we can dispose of the disgrace that their non-response caused.

- Help them discover their annoyance. Outrage is an extraordinarily versatile feeling, and it's one we don't permit ourselves to have. We think the outrage is terrible. However, outrage gives us where our sound limits were crossed.

Outrage gives us vitality to conquer the deterrent. We can help the patient see they had the enthusiastic vitality to survive, yet the vitality couldn't be shown at the time they needed it.

On the off chance that, in a meeting, we can get a patient to distinguish their annoyance, they will see that they were not totally inert to the awful accident. On the off chance that we can enable them to feel even the littlest development of a micro-expression of outrage all over - the slight downturn of the internal eyebrows - we can show them their body didn't thoroughly sell out them at that time.

We can reconnect their body and their sentiments to their feelings. This builds up a condition of consistency - where their inside sentiments coordinate their external exhibitions of those emotions.

Further, as a dissociative memory is investigated, discovering outrage and decreasing disgrace takes into account the memory to in a general sense change. Outrage brings them out of separation, regardless of whether it is outrage at you, the specialist!

- Introduce body development. Since shutdown makes us freeze, reactivating body developments while discussing the injury is an extraordinary method to reconnect the body and psyche, to bring them out of shutdown.

For instance, one of my patients was in a mishap. At the point when the EMS appeared, they lashed her to a gurney to stack her into the rear of a rescue vehicle. More than the genuine mishap, being caught on that gurney was horrendous for her. For the whole ride to the emergency clinic, she was startled that she'd hurt her neck, and the entirety of the tension that encompasses a neck injury made her be solidified in dread.

Indeed, even in discussing the injury in the treatment meeting, her body was firm, solidified, and she was separating.

I asked her, "How might you have needed to move during that minute?" She said she would have needed her arms to have the option to move. I asked her to gradually, carefully, move her arms in the manner in which she would have needed to.

It's critical to do the development carefully and gradually, concentrating on the vibe of the development. That patient felt an enormous arrival of vitality. In the accompanying meetings, she had the option to tell the memory as an account, rather than separating.

Having the patient move - slow punching, kicking, contorting, running set up - flips the individual from shutdown into the battle or flight mode, with the objective being to move into association, or social commitment, mode.

Body development works out, related to conversing with an advisor, can essentially change the memory.

- Practicing confidence. Enthusiastic shutdown can happen inside connections where one individual feels they can't speak with the other individual well.

One specialist, John Gottman, depicts this training as stonewalling. Rehearsing self-assuredness can help the patient feel more in charge of their passionate state, and have a sense of security to move into sound relationship designs.

- Breath-work, care, and yoga all have a job in getting increasingly associated with your present time and place body. I will examine this subject finally in a future digital broadcast.

Showing yourself how to all the more likely ensure yourself, later on, can be ground-breaking and furthermore resets the pressure framework after some time. I discussed quality preparing in an earlier scene, and later on, will discuss figuring out how to battle as a functioning method to not stay detached or an unfortunate casualty both in outlook and capacity. Further accomplishing something hard, on a progressing premise, considers building inward quality which can keep you in battle and flight longer before going into shut down.

CHAPTER FOUR: CHILDREN, EMOTIONAL REGULATION, AND POLYVAGAL THEORY

As Parents, our duty is to assist kids with handling through their encounters. This isn't a simple assignment. It is anything but difficult to feel activated by kids' huge feelings, regardless of whether it is dread, outrage, or pity; particularly when the declaration of these sentiments turns out as troublesome practices. The polyvagal theory enables Parents to explore your youngster's extremely enthusiastic states.

Kids may get resistant, decline to rest, begin lying, or become forceful with kin or Parents. As parents, it isn't unexpected to endeavor to apply outcomes or rebuff our youngsters. In any case, this can decline into a battle of will, where Parents would prefer not to be the first to yield. While limit setting is important to guard our kids and ourselves, it is basic that we help our kids loosen up their passionate dysregulation in the security of a mindful relationship.

Polyvagal Theory gives a neurobiological system to understanding the association between the brain, body, and feelings. Enabled with more profound comprehension, we increment our ability to sympathetically and effectively bolster youngsters' passionate guidelines.

Being a sentiments analyst

Youngsters need Adults to assist them with handling through their passionate reactions to the world; sentiments that happen during ordinary formative achievements and furthermore from upsetting or awful life occasions. There are times in parenting where you have to play the job of investigator to decide the reason for your kid's misery. Is it hunger, insufficient rest, tactile based, an adjustment in the schedule, kin elements, or an occasion that occurred at school?

As Parents, when we associate with youngsters who are dysregulated inwardly, we frequently feel upset as well. On the off chance that you see your kid feeling on edge almost certainly, you will feel stressed for your youngster and may even scrutinize your parenting aptitudes. On the off chance that a youngster is attempting to hit you, it is entirely expected to feel irate, frightful, or guarded. On the off chance that these practices happen all the time, you will create sentiments of disdain towards your kid. This doesn't mean you are an awful parent and it is essential to have apparatuses to react successfully to feelings as they emerge inside our kids and us.

Polyvagal theory and kids

Kids regularly experience issues conveying their sentiments verbally; therefore they much of the time express enthusiastic misery typically. A few kids will, in general, hold enormous sentiments inside. A portion of these kids pull back and abstain from associating with others. Other youngsters are progressively hazardous in nature. These kids may have irate upheavals, pitching sensational fits. In some cases, youngsters are forceful towards other relatives, and others may hurt themselves by pulling out hair or picking at skin. As Parents, these practices can be upsetting to find in kids. However, these practices are additionally techniques that kids use to control their psyche, body, and feelings.

Researches uncover that the elements of the autonomic sensory system are controlled by the vagus nerve in the body. The vagus nerve interfaces the brain to significant frameworks in the body including the stomach and gut, heart, lungs, throat, and facial muscles. Polyvagal theory sets that there are three parts of the vagus nerve; one liable for thoughtful activities, one reaction for parasympathetic activities, and the third, which intervenes and directs the activities of both called the social sensory system. How about we take a gander at these in more noteworthy detail:

- The social sensory system is related to association, tranquility, wellbeing, and attention on the present minute. This segment of the vagus nerve exhausts the face and is found in our children through shimmer in their eyes, a grin on their appearances, and trust in their capacity to move toward the world. The social sensory system is fortified by connections and helps kids effectively explore their thoughtful and parasympathetic sensory systems.

- The thoughtful sensory system is related with high excitement and preparation towards development. In youngsters, you can perceive thoughtful actuation when children are energized, senseless, keyed up, wiggly or squirmy, shocked, irate, on edge, or experience issues dozing. When feeling hazardous or compromised, this shows as a battle or flight reaction. Anyway, when upheld by the social sensory system, this enactment can prepare for the play.

- The parasympathetic sensory system is related to low excitement, unwinding, withdrawal or sadness. At the point when youngsters feel compromised, they may pull back, seem defenseless, and state they are worn out, exhausted, or miscrable. Anyway, when upheld by the social sensory system, kids have a sense of security to unwind into an embrace, cuddle with a pet, or wait in calm fulfilling exercises, for example, perusing or drawing.

As Parents, information on the polyvagal theory enables you to help the advancement of the social sensory system in kids to assist them with getting very much adjusted.

Spared by the ball

Here is an individual story that shows the procedure of how we can function with our own feelings to manage our kids:

Following a difficult day, I requested that the children get the toys in the lounge room. Neither one of the children was tuning in. Rather they started squabbling with one another, contending about who made the greater chaos. We were all bad-tempered. I had spent my rationale for the afternoon. I was feeling disappointment ascend inside me. I felt the motivation to holler. I took a full breath, glanced around, and afterward... the soccer ball made all the difference. Rather than taking my sentiments out on the children, I went to the ball and energetically stated,

"Soccer ball, you are not going into the crate! I am so irate with your soccer ball. You are not tuning in to me!" The children and I began chuckling at how senseless it was that I was shouting at the soccer ball and they requested that I do it once more! At that point, they began to tell the different toys that they weren't going on the racks either. We, at that point, cooperated in taking care of the toys, energetically contending with the toys concerning why they expected to head to sleep.

Tools for passionate guideline

The objective of passionate guidelines is to assist kids with realizing that they can have emotions and still be alright, safe, and adored. Here are a few apparatuses I prescribe for when your kid's practices are flagging enthusiastic trouble:

- Do a self-check first: In a plane, you get guidelines to put your breathing device on first; at that point, place it on your youngster. Accept this significant guidance. Ask yourself, would you say you are initiated? What manner of speaking would you say you are utilizing? What is your non-verbal communication conveying? What do you need at the present time? Perhaps you have to extend, inhale, or call somebody who can assist you with feeling progressively associated and safe. On the off chance that your kid's practices are putting themselves or any other individual in danger, by all methods address the worry right away. Yet, in addition, perceive that escaping from your kid is now and then the most ideal approach to protect both yourself and your kid. Self-guideline is testing; be that as it may, rehearsing your techniques before your kid gives important demonstrating. For instance, you may state, "Whew, I am feeling frantic at this moment! I will inhale and step my feet. Ahh, that feels much improved… "

- Become a feeling criminologist: Once you can be increasingly present, watch your kid's practices and be interested in which sensory system state is predominant. What is their non-verbal communication saying? What methodology is your kid utilizing right presently to oversee feelings? Would you be able to enable your youngster to encounter association? This will help fortify the social sensory system.

- High excitement apparatuses: If your kid is profoundly actuated, investigate meeting them in the high vitality in a steady, fun-loving style. This may include allowing them to push against you while you hold immovably onto a pad or utilizing rich swords to play battle. I generally tell kids that outrage is a solid feeling, and we have to locate a sound method to allow it to out. My child likes to hit a pad while he imparts his irate sentiments to me.

- Low excitement devices: If your kid is pulled back or close down, check whether they will permit you to come right up-front. Utilize your breath and voice tone to impart to your youngster that you give it a second thought. My little girl wants to cover up under a cover when she is overpowered. My activity in those minutes is to smoothly sit by her, just advising her that I am there. In the end, she will twist up on my lap, crucial.

When to look for proficient assistance

At the point when we are stuck in a dynamic with our kids that vibe unfortunate or reliably negative, it is an indication to look for more help. Once in a while, this is a sign to get more prominent comprehension about your kid's practices. On the off chance that your kid has progressing difficulties with sensory, animosity, or withdrawal you don't need to experience this by itself. There are likewise times that looking for more prominent symptomatic clearness is important to manage suitable mediations. Information and aptitudes just take us up until now, particularly when youngsters trigger us as Parents! One of my objectives as an analyst and essayist is to de-trash psycho-treatment. It tends to be lowering and agonizing over requesting help, inspired by a paranoid fear of being judged or seen as a terrible parent. Now and then, getting proficient help for ourselves and our kids is probably the best blessing we can give the people to come.

Are Children Naturally Resilient?

We need to confide in our kids' ability to deal with life's troubles and we would prefer not to over-secure them. In the event that we, as Parents, hop in too rapidly to take care of issues for our kids, we may prevent their capacity to build up their own critical thinking aptitudes. As youngsters figure out how to take care of issues, they build up their ability to be inventive and acknowledge they have an effect on their reality. The world we live in isn't constantly sheltered and kind and we have to have certainty that our kids can eventually deal with this defective world.

In any case, when kids have confronted a mind-boggling life occasion, they regularly need assistance preparing what they have seen and how they feel. At the point when a youngster faces stressors or difficulties, we would prefer not to over-gauge their capacity to deal with it all alone. The result of not supporting kids to process horrible accidents might be lost inventive, scholarly, or social potential.

"In a perfect world, we give youngsters the perfect measure of freedom and challenge offset with adequate help and wellbeing."

Bringing up Resilient Children

Flexibility is our capacity to adjust well even with misfortune; it signifies "bobbing back" from troublesome encounters. As a quality based therapist, I apply to inquire about versatility to my work with kids and families. Caring Adults bring up versatile kids by helping them to comprehend their lives and feel progressively skilled inside their social, passionate, and intellectual advancement.

As Parents, caring emotionally supportive networks assist us with getting to our flexibility so we can enable our youngsters to build up their strength. Versatile kids are sustained via caring Adults who can help them effectively express their experience.

- Younger youngsters may better communicate through play or drawing their involvement in a mindful Adult.

- Older youngsters profit by discussions that reflect feelings, investigate troublesome choices, and inspect the implications kids make about their encounters.

At the point when Children throw you a Curve Ball

Being with a kid who is battling leads most Parents to feel irate or terrified. Particularly when:

- "My kid won't rest or stay unconscious!"
- "My child is forceful and is hitting his more youthful sister or me!"
- "My little girl used to go to class fine and dandy and now she sticks and won't discrete from me when I drop her off for first grade!"
- "My youngster is blocking me out and simply doesn't hear me out!"

Now and then we respond or close down our kids due to our feelings of trepidation and awkward feelings. To need to push our youngsters away or flee from our kids is an ordinary and organically determined reaction when we are apprehensive. Be that as it may, I welcome you to see your kid's "curveballs" as a call to draw in your kid, to look underneath the conduct, and to associate with their inward world.

Realizing that you now and then experience outrage when you are defenseless and apprehensive can help you brilliantly turn towards your kid's troublesome practices that emerge out of their vulnerabilities and fears.

Strength is for Parents Too

For Parents, strength permits us to react imaginatively to the difficulties inborn in bringing up our youngsters. Parents need support through merciful associations with accomplices, different Parents, and when fundamental, advisors, to assist us with investigating the more profound topics of responses to youngsters and how this might be associated with the past. Being a strong parent

Implies:

- Getting backing to gain from your deterrents so you can bolster your kids to gain from their battles.
- Accepting that you are blemished so you can be kinder towards your kids' errors.
- Recognizing that you don't have all the appropriate responses with the goal that you are additionally tolerating when kids feel lost or befuddled.
- Remembering that you like being adored and known for what your identity is so you can expect to love and know your youngsters for what their identity is.

On a plane, they will consistently advise the Adults to put their breathing apparatus on first – at that point, help your youngster to put theirs on. The equivalent is valid with versatility: When Adults feel bolstered they are better ready to help their kids.

Strength Informed Treatment

As individuals, we would all be able to get "stuck" in some cases. There is no compelling reason to feel embarrassed or humiliated to request help, whether it is for yourself or your youngster. Flexibility educated treatment perceives that when Parents and youngsters have a sense of security and bolstered you can get to your innovativeness, quality, and ability to deal with life's difficulties.

CHAPTER FIVE: POLYVAGAL THEORY AND ANXIETY

Polyvagal Theory may give inventive intercessions to both tension and wretchedness. Numerous individuals become caught in ruminating about the past or agonizing over the future; they can't appear to keep their brain and body right now. Some solid, dread based, real resistances may not react well to "talk treatment" alone. In helping customers with such enduring, it is critical to incorporate an exceptionally solid clinical collusion and relationship, just as close to home story on interior introjected messages about their vulnerabilities, fears, and self-questions. Review that uneasiness is commonly a body-based safeguard from lower brain territories (limbic and mind stem). These territories are regularly un-influenced when simply "talk" happens in treatment. There are sure signs that an individual's tension is misbehaving in a clinical meeting. These are:

- Higher pitched voice, now and then with quick conveyance;
- Prolonged hushes;
- Tighter, level face and tight jaw – regularly with the upper cosmetic touch-ups marginally;
- Random apprehensive body developments;
- Rapid, higher-chest relaxing;
- Problems in mindfulness, memory, and subjective appreciation; and,
- Sometimes out and out frenzy.

At the point when such restless resistances show up, the advisor needs to move to establish and quiet breathing mediations. Talking it through, working it through might be lacking to reestablish feeling guidelines. It is recommended to initiate polyvagal impedance to uneasiness. In the event that effective, feeling guidelines will be restored.

- Request the customer to breathe out more gradually, and with more accentuation.
- Then have the individual expand their exhalation marginally. Be mindful so as not to

- expand excessively far; inconvenience will follow.
- If the individual is frightful of open talking or introducing in a gathering treatment meeting, demand that they add more words to their sentences. This will require an adjustment in breathing procedure – consequently expanding the exhalation.
- Practice longer exhalations as the customer inhales all the more gradually and all the more profoundly.
- Have the customer lay on their back with their marginally bowed legs high up on a divider – relax

At the point when your body encounters uneasiness, it does what it's prepared to do: respond to the condition of dread you're detecting.

As Stephen Porges says, "Uneasiness is our higher mind structures deciphering a substantial (lower brain) reaction as requiring a guard."

In case you're acquainted with uneasiness or stress, you realize the heart dashing, chest-beating and real dread that ascents like a flee lift in your body. It can forget about you lashing with fury and outrage or leaving your prompt condition as everything whirls into an awkward blend of overpowering.

Instructing yourself to unwind once in a while works

Tuning in to other people who let you know not to stress seldom works either.

How Your Body Responds To Stress and Anxiety

At the point when your mind detects fear, it actuates your thoughtful sensory system. Everything alerts, alarms and glimmering lights are making your body aware of threat ... regardless of whether the 'risk' is by and large late for a significant gathering, contending with your accomplice, or attempting to make it to take a shot at time subsequent to managing an agitated youngster.

At the point when these alerts go off you'll see these physiological changes as blood is coordinated to parts of the body important to deal with the apparent threat:

- You're breathing shifts more into the upper piece of your chest
- Your breaths become shorter
- Your pulse rises
- Your muscles become progressively tense
- The upper piece of your face becomes compliment or has less appearance
- Your voice turns out to be all the more piercing with a smaller scope of pitch

When the risk is over your body's parasympathetic sensory system restores your body to its harmony. Furthermore, life goes on … until the following upsetting occasion happens - OR the pressure you're encountering in your life is all inescapable and accordingly is keeping your body on high alarm in any event when there is no 'activating' occurrence for you to feel on edge.

Why Your Personal Narrative Adds To The Problem

As your body moves into an on edge state, what you enlighten yourself concerns the importance behind the inclination matters.

For instance, you might be:

- Telling yourself that you're dreadful of getting into a lift, an airplane or a room without windows as it triggers considerations of a past horrible mishap
- Avoiding swarmed places or boisterous situations as they trigger overpower
- Hearing your internal identity recommend things that could not be right in the event that you see your chief/supervisor strolling towards you (for example I've committed an error, I'll be sacked, somebody's griped about me, I've been late for gatherings)
- Noticing your child or little child waking and feeling overpowered at adapting to their vitality level, crying or not having the

- opportunity to finish the horde of things you have to do.
- Having dreams that wake you making you feel as though you're having a wellbeing emergency

These individual stories might be driving you to feel excessively incredulous of yourself, accusing yourself, feeling a feeling of disgrace or making a decision about yourself as basically 'not sufficient'.

Passionate states activated by tension are not intentional; they're customized from a transformative point of view. Your brain is ensuring you such that's protected warm-blooded creatures from the most punctual of times - it's a programmed reaction exuding from the most established piece of your mind - frequently called the reptilian mind.

Once 'risk' is felt, those 'on edge' reactions swell all through your body - implying that if your heart begins beating different pieces of your body (lungs, gut, muscles) will likewise 'get the dread message' and react.

In the event that you can figure out how to change one part of this automatic gradually expanding influence, at that point, it's conceivable to restore the body back to quiet more rapidly.

While it's not all that simple to slow your pulse (except if you're a rehearsed meditator) you can deal with your relaxing.

This is the reason why this method is basic, yet so compelling

To change your physiological state so you have a progressively positive, controlled and fitting reaction, it is recommended: controlling your breath.

While this method depends on conventional breathing activities, he makes it one stride further by presenting 'deceiving' your psyche into easing back you are relaxing.

He says: When you're encountering pressure, your hands and chest might be fixing. You're breathing from a higher point in your chest. Furthermore, these body reactions are making a physiological expression that underpins the sentiment of sensoryness.

Right now, the brain isn't preparing the coherent answer of 'simply unwind' on the grounds that you're encapsulating uneasiness and not taking in the meaningful gestures that could ease on edge sentiments.

While encountering a condition of pressure or tension, higher-request thinking gets restricted. In the event that somebody is encountering sensoryness, they may confuse an individual with an 'unbiased' demeanor all over as being undermining or potentially judgemental.

So figuring out how to oversee tension at the time is a significant aptitude to ace as your 'legitimate mind' can't bolster you in the manner in which it ordinarily does.

Breathing Technique:

Utilize this method to 'stunt' yourself into hindering your relaxing.

Breath out gradually by expanding the term of your expressions - for example: saying more words before slowly inhaling. He says that numerous individuals encountering tension change their discourse example and slowly inhale on each other word, so by taking more time to breathe out, you'll help your body's parasympathetic reaction (the piece of your autonomic framework that urges you to rest and unwind).

This is an incredible tip in case you're going to introduce at a gathering or give a discussion and need to quiet the nerves; however, shouldn't something be said about the ordinary circumstance?

An Every Day Breathing Technique You Can Use Anywhere

I like to utilize a comparative methodology, yet with an increasingly programmed technique - tallying.

It includes tallying in reverse from ten to one.

As you start, say the word 'ten' as gradually as possible, discharging your breath completely.

Presently take an ordinary breath in.

Now proceed with 'nine', saying it as gradually as you can and discharging your breath completely.

Proceed right now you reach 'one' - notice the distinction in your chest, gut region, shoulders, hands, facial muscles, throat and leg muscles.

Elective: For each number, picture the relating measure of candles. As you state each number, picture smothering the candles in a gradual breathe out. This diverts you from the wellspring of tension, so you center more on your breathing and extinguishing the candles.

CHAPTER SIX:
POLYVAGAL THEORY AND PTSD

One of the difficult repercussions of Post-Traumatic Stress Disorder (PTSD) is the experience of an absence of control that can happen when you feel caught by sentiments of sensoryness, alarm, overpower, or despair. Polyvagal theory, offers a significant system for comprehension and adequately reacting to the extraordinary passionate and physiological manifestations of PTSD.

"Mending the sensory system can require some investment and requires persistence. Put the polyvagal theory without hesitation in your life to expand your feeling of opportunity in body and brain" - Dr. Arielle Schwartz

The Sensory System: A Basic Model

An essential model of the sensory system shows that we have two segments of our sensory system, one that is under our cognizant control (for example moving your hand) and another that capacities without our mindfulness (for example controlling our internal heat level), the segment of the sensory system that capacity without our cognizant mindfulness is known as the autonomic sensory system (ANS). The entirety of our enthusiastic articulations are interceded by the ANS as it either activates vitality through our thoughtful sensory system or rations vitality through our parasympathetic sensory system.

- The thoughtful sensory system is related to the battle or flight reaction and the arrival of cortisol (stress synthetic substances) all through the circulatory system.
- The parasympathetic is related to unwinding, processing, and recovery.

The thoughtful and parasympathetic sensory systems are intended to work in a cadenced shift that underpins sound absorption, rest, and resistant framework working.

Modern researches offer a propelled comprehension of the ANS, particularly as identified with injury and PTSD. The autonomic sensory system is directed by the vagus nerve or the tenth cranial nerve. The vagus nerve interfaces the brain to significant frameworks in the body, supporting psyche body correspondences.

Warm-blooded animals have two vagal circuits, a developmentally more established circuit called the dorsal vagal intricate and an all the more as of late advanced vagal circuit called the "ventral vagal complex" (VVC) which is additionally alluded to as the "social sensory system." The dorsal vagal complex interfaces with the organs underneath the stomach, including the spleen, liver, kidneys, just as the little and internal organs. The ventral vagal, social sensory system interfaces over the stomach to your heart, lungs, larynx, pharynx, internal ear, just as the facial muscles around your mouth and eyes.

Extensively, the vagus nerve is constantly connected with the parasympathetic sensory system and has an inhibitory impact upon the heart and thoughtful sensory system movement. In particular, deeper examinations recognized that the parasympathetic sensory system has two introductions that rely on whether you have a sense of security or feel compromised. In the midst of security, the parasympathetic sensory system encourages rest, unwinding, and processing. In any case, in the midst of danger, the parasympathetic sensory system has a protective mode.

Bioconductal Defenses

At the point when we feel compromised, we will commonly endeavor to draw in the social sensory system to restore a feeling of association and security. On the off chance that we can't make protected, social security, we will logically fall back on developmentally more established bioconductal resistance techniques. In the first place, we will draw upon thoughtful sensory system activities, for example, battle or trip to prepare us into self-security. Here, you may feel temperamental, on edge, or panicky.

On the off chance that the thoughtful sensory system is ineffective in re-establishing security, we will default to the developmentally most seasoned piece of the vagus nerve, the "dorsal vagal complex"

(DVC). This increasingly crude technique connects with the parasympathetic sensory system in a foul way. Here, the parasympathetic sensory system connects with immobilizing cautious procedures, for example, separation or blacking out. Here, you may feel worn out, dazed, or sick.

The Vagal Brake

Both the dorsal vagal complex (DVC) and the ventral vagal complex (VVC) will apply hindrance to the thoughtful sensory system. The Polyvagal Theory utilizes an analogy proposing that the vagus nerve resembles squeezing the brake pedal when driving a vehicle. Expulsion of the parasympathetic "vagal brake" causes an expansion in pulse and more prominent helplessness to push.

The social sensory system works as a refined brake, which has quieting and alleviating impacts reflected in musical motions in pulse fluctuation. This is related to increments in wellbeing and enthusiastic prosperity. Conversely, the dorsal vagal complex acts as a sudden vagal brake. Stalling out right now a protective technique for significant stretches of time can have genuine repercussions on mental and physical wellbeing.

The Social Sensory System

Your social sensory system (VVC) is reinforced by myelination. Myelination is a greasy covering on nerve pathways that are expanded through rehashed use and results in speed up and control. You can envision here the myelination that happens in the learning of another bit of music for the piano. At first, notes are played gradually and cautiously; however, with rehashed practice, you start to make music, in the end without perusing the music by any stretch of the imagination. In like manner, the pathways of the social sensory system are reinforced through rehashed practice. You realize that you are in your social sensory system when you feel a glow in your grin and see the radiance in your eyes.

You can draw in your social sensory system to associate with others, feel fun-loving, and unwind into an association. On the off chance that you feel pointlessly keyed up with tension, you can utilize the social sensory system to distinguish that you are protected. You can glance around and tune in for signals of wellbeing or participate in systems, for example, quiet, slow breathing to enable you to unwind. These activities utilize the activity frameworks over the stomach.

When you realize that you are protected, you never again need to concentrate outward. This permits you to interface with the helpful side of your Dorsal Vagal Complex. Here, you can decide to immobilize into an encounter of security by unwinding into an embrace with a friend or family member or resting into a sustaining contemplation. It is additionally conceivable to mix your social sensory system with your thoughtful sensory system, which encourages your capacity to participate in a vivacious play.

Your social sensory system expands your capacity to react successfully when you grope keyed with tension or shut-down with melancholy.

Activation into Play – Immobilization into Intimacy

Regardless of whether you are feeling uneasiness or melancholy, you can utilize instruments to draw in your social sensory system to restore higher request sensory system capacities.

On the off chance that you are encountering tension, you are likely in battle or flight, a key protection response of the thoughtful sensory system. Thoughtful activities include activation; the need to move your body to discharge the work of pressure cortisols. You can draw in your social apprehensive by scouring your hands together overwhelmingly and reaching to your own face, neck, upper chest, arms, and legs. You can likewise investigate physical developments that vibe safe and establishing, for example, taking a walk or shaking your arms and legs to discharge pressure. At the point when we have a sense of security, we can connect with our social sensory system to utilize the vitality of the thoughtful sensory system to move, play, and giggle.

Feeling shut down, crumbled, discouraged, or numb means that you are in the cautious responses of your parasympathetic sensory system which is portrayed by immobilization. In the event that you have a background marked by injury, it is conceivable that you are seeing dangers in your condition that are not really happening in the present time and place. This is on the grounds that a typical indication of PTSD is disarray between the past and the present. Right now, the social sensory system can help perceive that you are not in fast approaching peril. This permits you to get to the positive, loosening up components of your parasympathetic sensory system to "rest and review." When conceivable, turn towards a caring association with a companion, caring accomplice, or a pet. At first, you may need to look or call somebody you trust and tune in to the sound of their voice. You can likewise imagine a caring creature, companion, or defensive partner to reestablish a felt feeling of association.

At the point when you can grasp immobilization with security, you can get to the sustenance of the unwinding reaction.

Suggestions for Healing PTSD

The polyvagal theory in real life can permit you to expand your feeling of opportunity in body and brain while encountering manifestations of tension, frenzy, or sadness. Here are a few recommendations:

- Focus on the present minute
- Engage the feeling of smell with basic oil that brings a positive affiliation or feeling
- Re-set up association by calling a companion, cuddling with your pet, or cherishing self-touch
- Express emotions through talking, composing, drawing, or development
- Focus on your breath as a calibrating instrument to control the sensory system
- Engage in care practice, for example, reflection or remedial yoga
- Allow yourself to play or get innovative
- Focus on the great by tuning into the magnificence around you

Restorative ramifications of Polyvagal Theory educate Somatic brain science and EMDR

Treatment. Recuperating the sensory system can require some serious energy and requires persistence with the procedure and with yourself. You are not bombing when you feel on edge or discouraged. You are additionally not the only one. Put the polyvagal theory vigorously in your life to build your feeling of opportunity in the body and brain. Further Reading:

Recuperating from Developmental Trauma

Awful encounters are, by their very definition, terrifying and overpowering. Occasions such as auto collisions, catastrophic events, or demonstrations of brutality, change our natural direction to the world. It isn't unexpected to feel overflowed with incredible feelings, sensations, or recollections as we adjust to new and frequently undesirable reality. Some of the time we begin to maintain a strategic distance from places suggestive of the injury. Or on the other hand, we may have or have nosy recollections and emotions. Post-Traumatic Stress Disorder (PTSD) alludes to the nearness of these indications well after the occasion is finished. Nonetheless, Complex

PTSD and separation is another sort of post awful pressure.

At the point when you experience youth disregard or constant maltreatment, your essential direction to the world is one of danger, dread, and endurance. Deceitful Parents or parental figures leave you untrusting or befuddled about what comprises a caring relationship. Dread and absence of security leaves you checking your condition for potential dangers. An ignored or mishandled kid will depend upon worked in, organic assurance components for endurance to "block out" the risk. Examples of dread and separation advise the creating body and psyche.

"Adults mishandled as youngsters frequently report feeling vulnerable, sad, despair, profound dejection, disgrace, shamefulness, bad form, clearing discouragement, and self-destructive musings. Many keep on pushing the unnerving, yucky, difficult, and confounding emotions far away by turning to learned dissociative examples. Despite the fact that you are protected now, it can feel overpowering to recognize leftovers of verifiable dangers held in the body, feelings, and brain. We mend early formative injury inside a protected relationship that is conscious, unsurprising, predictable, non-guarded and has clear limits. Delicately we rethink our ability for a relationship with a dependable other. Gradually we reconstruct confidence in ourselves."

Separation and Defenses

Kids require consistency and normality with parental figures so they can grow clear assumptions regarding themselves and the world. Such steadiness gives the ground of security and permits kids to adjust to the internal changes that normally happen during early improvement. When stood up to with a perilous and unusual condition, babies and youngsters block out and go off to endure. Separation turns into a very much kept up division between the piece of oneself engaged with staying aware of everyday undertakings of living and those parts that are holding the feelings of dread, disgrace, or outrage.

Dissociative side effects can be generally mellow, for example, feeling foggy or fluffy, making some hard memories discussing encounters, feeling mixed up, and feeling tired. Increasingly extreme side effects incorporate inclination "crazy," having breaches of memory, or reports of "lost time." In the most serious circumstances of Dissociative Identity Disorder, it is conceivable to build up various parts with unmistakable sub-characters.

Complex PTSD and separation are kept up by barriers, for example, refusal, constraint, romanticizing, or minimization of the past. Or then again, we use substances or keep up other addictive practices to abstain from feeling the agony. Here are a few models:

- "Yeah, he was an abuser; however, it is anything but a serious deal."
- "They were awesome Parents; however, they celebrated a great deal and I was left to raise myself a significant part of the time."
- "It's simply an excessive amount to recognize what occurred."
- "Why feel when I can… eat, drink, smoke pot, take a valium, and so on."

Settling Complex PTSD and Dissociation

Horrendous examples will, in general, be remembered and re-sanctioned. Despite the fact that they are agonizing, horrendous examples are commonplace; giving up can really feel additionally overpowering. It can feel more secure not to confide in individuals. It can feel simpler not to change.

Social psycho-treatment with a clinician educated about a formative injury can help. Suggested modalities incorporate EMDR Treatment and Somatic Treatment (body-focused). Scientists propose that the recuperating of early formative injury must happen inside a sheltered relationship that is aware, unsurprising, reliable, non-protective, and that has clear limits. The way toward mending complex PTSD includes:

- Observing your examples of separation.
- Accepting and adoring yourself with the entirety of your barriers.
- Compassionately perceiving the effect of separation on your life and connections today.

- Recognizing that an awful accident transpired.
- Realizing that expanded mindfulness brings expanded decision.
- Increasing resilience for dismissal, misfortune, disillusionment, disgrace, strife, and vulnerability.
- Decreasing the dependence upon guards that keep up a separation from difficult sentiments.
- Recognizing that the startling or risky occasions are over at this point.
- Distinguishing between the over a wide span of time all the more unmistakably.
- Reclaiming adaptability in your body and psyche.
- Developing new, solid assumptions regarding connections.
- Having an away from the effect of social injuries experienced in youth develops empathy.

Developing Compassion

Regardless of whether you are a customer, a clinician, a mindful companion, or an accomplice, having an away from the effect of youth social injury develops sympathy. Adults manhandled as kids can feel vulnerability, misery, despair, profound forlornness, disgrace, shamefulness, bad form, clearing despondency, and self-destructive musings. Many keep on pushing the alarming, yucky, difficult, and befuddling emotions far away by turning to learned dissociative examples.

Numerous individuals with a background marked by complex PTSD and separation have been misconstrued, misdiagnosed, and over-cured. Shockingly, good-natured care-suppliers can accept that side effects are the aftereffect of a shortcoming of character; a harming outcome that "accuses the person in question" and meddles with recuperating.

Despite the fact that there might be security now, it can even now feel overpowering to recognize the remainders of chronicled dangers held in body, feelings, and brain. Tenderly recuperating happens in a relationship with a reliable other. Gradually we revamp confidence in ourselves.

CHAPTER SEVEN:
THE VAGAL PARADOX

The gauge of vagal tone got from estimating respiratory sinus arrhythmia, could be utilized in clinical medicine as a record of pressure defenselessness. Instead of utilizing the engaging proportions of pulse changeability (i.e., beat-to-thump fluctuation) as often as possible utilized in obstetrics and pediatrics, the paper underlined that respiratory sinus arrhythmia has neural inception and speaks to the tonic utilitarian outpouring from the vagus to the heart (i.e., cardiovascular vagal tone). Along these lines, it was recommended that respiratory sinus arrhythmia would give a more delicate file of wellbeing status than an increasingly worldwide proportion of beat-to-thump pulse fluctuation reflecting unsure neural and nonneural systems.

The paper introduced a quantitative methodology that applied time-arrangement investigations to separate the abundancy of respiratory sinus arrhythmia as a progressively exact list of vagal action. The article gave information showing that sound full-term newborn children had respiratory sinus arrhythmia of essentially more noteworthy abundancy than did preterm babies. This thought of utilizing pulse examples to record vagal action was not new, having been accounted for as right on time as 1910 by Hering.5 Moreover, contemporary examinations have dependably detailed that vagal bar through atropine discourages respiratory sinus arrhythmia in warm-blooded animals.

A neonatologist, as a clinical understudy, discovered that vagal tone could be deadly. He contended that might be an overdose of something that is otherwise good (i.e., vagal tone) could be terrible. He was alluding, obviously, to the clinical danger of neurogenic bradycardia. Bradycardia, when seen during conveyance, might be a pointer of fetal misery. Thus, bradycardia and apnea are significant pointers of hazard for the infant.

Further examination were done on this bewildering perception by considering the human baby during conveyance. Fetal bradycardia happened just when respiratory sinus arrhythmia was discouraged (i.e., a respiratory beat in the fetal pulse is perceptible even without the enormous chest divider developments related to breathing that happen postpartum). This brought up the issue of how vagal instruments could intercede both respiratory sinus arrhythmia and bradycardia, as one is defensive and the other is conceivably deadly. This irregularity turned into the "vagal oddity" and filled in as the inspiration driving the polyvagal theory.

With respect to the instruments intervening bradycardia and pulse inconstancy, there is a conspicuous irregularity among information and physiological suspicions. Physiological models expect vagal guidelines of both chronotropic control of the heart (i.e., pulse) and the abundancy of respiratory sinus arrhythmia. For instance, it has been dependably detailed that vagal cardio-inhibitory filaments to the heart have steady utilitarian properties portrayed by bradycardia to neural incitement and respiratory rhythm.[9] However, despite the fact that there are circumstances where the two measures covary (e.g., during exercise and cholinergic barricade), there are different circumstances in which the measures seem to reflect autonomous wellsprings of neural control (e.g., bradycardic scenes related with hypoxia, vasovagal syncope, and fetal trouble). As opposed to these detectable marvels, scientists keep on arguing for covariation between these two parameters. This irregularity, in light of a suspicion of a solitary focal vagal source, is the thing that I have marked the vagal Catch.

Examination of the phylogeny of the vertebrate autonomic sensory system gives a response to the vagal Catch. Research in near neuroanatomy and neurophysiology has distinguished two parts of the vagus, with each branch supporting distinctive versatile capacities and social systems. The vagal yield to the heart from one branch is showed in respiratory sinus arrhythmia, and the yield from the other branch is showed in bradycardia and perhaps the more slow rhythms in pulse changeability. In spite of the fact that the more slow rhythms have been expected to have a thoughtful impact, they are obstructed by atropine.

The polyvagal theory, explains how every one of three phylogenetic stages in the improvement of the vertebrate autonomic sensory system is related to a particular autonomic subsystem that is held and communicated in warm-blooded creatures. These autonomic subsystems are phylogenetically requested and typically connected to social correspondence (e.g., outward appearance, vocalization, tuning in), assembly (e.g., battle flight practices), and immobilization (e.g., faking passing, vasovagal syncope, and conduct shutdown).

The social correspondence framework (i.e., social commitment framework; see underneath) includes the myelinated vagus, which serves to encourage quiet conduct states by restraining thoughtful impacts to the heart and hosing the hypothalamic-pituitary-adrenal (HPA) axis. The assembly framework is subject to the working of the thoughtful sensory system. The most phylo-hereditarily crude segment, the immobilization framework, is subject to the unmyelinated vagus, which is imparted to most vertebrates. With expanded neural unpredictability coming about because of phylogenetic improvement, the creature's conduct and full of feeling collection is advanced. The three circuits can be conceptualized as unique, giving versatile reactions to sheltered, hazardous, and dangerous occasions and settings.

Just warm-blooded creatures have a myelinated vagus. In contrast to the unmyelinated vagus, starting in the dorsal engine core of the vagus with pre-and postganglionic muscarinic receptors, the mammalian myelinated vagus begins in the core ambiguous and has preganglionic nicotinic receptors and postganglionic muscarinic receptors. The unmyelinated vagus is imparted to different vertebrates, including reptiles, creatures of land and water, teleosts, and elasmobranchs.

We are presently examining the chance of extricating various highlights of the pulse example to progressively screen the two vagal frameworks. Starter concentrates in our research center to help this chance. In these investigations, we have hindered the nicotinic preganglionic receptors with hexamethonium and the muscarinic receptors with atropine. The information was gathered from the prairie vole, which has a high surrounding vagal tone. This primer information showed that, in a few creatures, nicotinic bar specifically evacuates respiratory sinus arrhythmia without hosing the adequacy of the lower frequencies in pulse inconstancy. Conversely, hindering the muscarinic receptors with atropine evacuates both the low and respiratory frequencies.

Consistency with Jacksonian Dissolution

The three circuits are sorted out and react to difficulties in a phylogenetically decided chain of importance reliable with the Jacksonian standard of disintegration. Jackson suggested that in the brain, higher (i.e., phylogenetically more up to date) neural circuits hinder lower (i.e., phylogenetically more seasoned) neural circuits and "when the higher are unexpectedly rendered functionless, the lower ascend in activity." Although Jackson proposed disintegration to clarify changes in mind work because of harm and ailment, the polyvagal theory proposes a comparable phylogenetically requested various leveled model to portray the grouping of autonomic reaction systems to challenges.

Practically, when nature is seen as protected, two significant highlights are communicated. Real state is controlled in a proficient way to advance development and reclamation (e.g., instinctive homeostasis). This is done through an expansion in the impact of mammalian myelinated vagal engine pathways on the cardiovascular pacemaker that eases back the heart, restrains the battle flight instruments of the thoughtful sensory system, hoses the pressure reaction arrangement of the HPA pivot (e.g., cortisol), and decreases aggravation by balancing resistant responses (e.g., cytokines). Second, through the procedure of development, the brainstem cores that manage the myelinated vagus got incorporated with the cores that direct the muscles of the face and head.

This connection brings about the bidirectional coupling between unconstrained social commitment practices and real states. In particular, an incorporated social commitment framework developed in warm-blooded animals when the neural guideline of instinctive states that advance development and reclamation (by means of the myelinated vagus) was connected neuroanatomically and neurophysiologically with the neural guideline of the muscles controlling eye stare, outward appearance, tuning in, and prosody.

The human sensory system, like that of different warm-blooded animals, developed not exclusively to make due in safe conditions yet additionally to advance endurance in perilous and dangerous settings. To achieve this versatile adaptability, the human sensory system held two progressively crude neural circuits to manage guarded techniques (i.e., battle flight and passing pretending practices). Note that social conduct, social correspondence, and instinctive homeostasis are contradictory to the neurophysiological states and practices advanced by the two neural circuits that help barrier systems. Therefore, by means of advancement, the human sensory system holds three neural circuits, which are in a phylogenetically sorted out chain of command. Right now, versatile reactions, the most up to date circuit is utilized first; if that circuit neglects to give wellbeing, the more established circuits are selected successively.

Examination of the phylogeny of the vertebrate heart has prompted extraction of four rules that give a premise to testing of speculations relating specific neural components to social commitment, battle flight, and passing pretending practices:

- There is a phylogenetic move in the guideline of the heart from endocrine correspondence to unmyelinated nerves, lastly to myelinated nerves.

- There is an advancement of contradicting neural components of excitation and restraint to give a fast guideline of evaluated metabolic yield.

- A face - heart association developed as source cores of vagal pathways moved ventrally from the more established dorsal engine core to the core ambiguous. This brought about an anatomical and neurophysiological linkage between neural guidelines of the heart by means of the myelinated vagus and the exceptional instinctive efferent pathways that control the striated muscles of the face and head, framing an incorporated social commitment framework.

- With expanded cortical improvement, the cortex shows more noteworthy power over the brainstem by means of direct (e.g., corticobulbar) and backhanded (e.g., corticoreticular) neural pathways beginning in engine cortex and ending in the source cores of the myelinated engine nerves rising up out of the brainstem (e.g., specific neural pathways inserted inside cranial nerves V, VII, IX, X, and XI), controlling visceromotor structures (i.e., heart, bronchi) just as somatomotor structures (muscles of the face and head).

Neuroception: Contextual Cueing of Adaptive, Maladaptive Physiological States

Too successfully change from guarded to social commitment methodologies, the mammalian sensory system needs to perform two significant versatile errands:

- Valuate hazard, and
- If the earth is seen as protected, hinder the more crude limbic structures that control battle, flight, or freeze practices.

Any boost that has the potential for expanding a creature's understanding of security has the capability of selecting the developmentally further developed neural circuits that help the prosocial practices of the social commitment framework.

The sensory system, through the handling of tactile data from nature and from the viscera, consistently assesses hazards. Since the neural assessment of hazard doesn't require cognizant mindfulness and may include subcortical limbic structures, the term neuroception22 was acquainted with stress a neural procedure, particularly from observation, that is equipped for recognizing ecological (and instinctive) highlights that are sheltered, hazardous, or perilous. In save situations, the autonomic state is adaptively managed to hose thoughtful actuation and to ensure the oxygen-subordinate focal sensory system, particularly the cortex, from the metabolic traditionalist responses of the dorsal vagal complex. In any case, how does the sensory system know when the earth is sheltered, perilous, or hazardous, and which neural instruments assess this hazard?

Ecological segments of neuroception

Neuroception speaks to a neural procedure that empowers people and different warm-blooded animals to participate in social practices by recognizing safe from hazardous settings. Neuroception is proposed as a conceivable component intervening both the demeanor and the disturbance of positive social conduct, feeling guideline, and instinctive homeostasis. Neuroception may be activated by include finders including regions of the worldly cortex that speak with the focal core of the amygdala and the periaqueductal dark since limbic reactivity is tweaked by fleeting cortex reactions to the expectation of voices, faces, and hand developments. In this manner, the neuroception of comfortable people and people with suitably prosodic voices and warm, expressive appearances converts into social communication advancing a feeling of security.

In many people (i.e., those without a mental issue or neuropathology), the sensory system assesses risks and matches the neurophysiological state with the genuine danger of the earth. At the point when nature is assessed as being sheltered, the guarded limbic structures are restrained, empowering social commitment and quiet instinctive states to develop. Interestingly, a few people experience befuddle and the sensory system assesses nature as being hazardous in any event, when it is protected. This befuddle brings about physiological states that help battle, flight, or freeze practices, yet not social commitment practices. As per the theory, social correspondence can be communicated effectively through the social commitment framework just when these protective circuits are restrained.

Different supporters of neuroception

The highlights of hazard in nature don't exclusively drive neuroception. Afferent input from the viscera gives a significant middle person of the availability of prosocial circuits related to social commitment practices. For instance, the polyvagal theory predicts that conditions of the assembly would bargain with our capacity to distinguish positive expressive gestures. Practically, instinctive states shading our view of articles and others. In this way, similar highlights of one individual drawing in another may bring about a scope of results, contingent upon the physiological condition of the objective person. In the event that the individual being locked in will be in a state wherein the social commitment framework is effectively available, equal prosocial collaborations are probably going to happen. Be that as it may, if the individual is in a condition of preparation, the equivalent drawing accordingly may be reacted to with the asocial highlights of withdrawal or animosity.

In such a state, it may be hard to hose the preparation circuit and empower the social commitment framework to return online.

The insula might be associated with the intervention of neuroception since it has been proposed as a mind structure engaged with passing on the diffuse criticism from the viscera into cognitive-mindfulness. Utilitarian imaging tests have exhibited that the insula assumes a significant job in the experience of agony and the experience of a few feelings, including outrage, dread, disturb, bliss, and pity. Critchley suggests that interior body states are spoken to in the insula and add to conditions of emotional inclination, and he has exhibited that action in the insula connects with interoceptive exactness.

CHAPTER EIGHT: DORSAL VAGAL, FREEZE, AND POLYVAGAL SOLUTIONS

As we talked about in the previous chapter, the essential job of the dorsal vagal framework, in people, is to manage organs beneath the stomach. In any case, that is by all accounts, not the only job. We should place it in context. Hereditarily, the dorsal vagal pathway of the autonomic sensory system is fundamentally the same as what's been seen in hard fish and even cartilaginous fish. When it developed to warm-blooded animals, its job was truly consigned fundamentally to beneath the stomach.

This implies it manages essentially every one of those instinctive organs that we are truly not mindful of. In any case, there are a few tracks, or pathways, that are still, as it were minimal, old frameworks that go to the heart and to zones like the throat. If you somehow managed to animate the uttermost, most profound piece of your throat, that would be controlled by the dorsal vagus. Obviously, what occurs in the event that you invigorate that piece of the throat? You disgorge

Disgorging is, one might say is a dorsal vagal reaction. The framework is truly going down and this is a versatile methodology for disposing of poisons and different things that might be happening. In any case, when we talk about the dorsal vagal framework it begins in the mind stem region called the dorsal engine core of the vagus or all the more generally now known as the dorsal core of the vagus.

A portion of the pathways really relocate through the core questionable and afterward return through the vagus and a portion of those that moved really wind up being a piece of the core equivocal or the ventral vagus. When you see it originating from the brain stem, you essentially have a bound together coordinated nerve. Many individuals feel that they're two separate nerves, the ventral vagus and the dorsal vagus; nonetheless, they're actually across the board conductor and we need to imagine that.

There are just about 15% of the filaments in that course. 15% to 20% of those strands are really efferent filaments significance going down from the mind. Of that 15%, really 80% of those are heading off to the dorsal vagus, and not many are setting off to the ventral vagus. So extremely, the prevalent highlights of our vagal framework are really managing sub-diaphragmatic organs. The significant part that we truly need to get to when we start talking about pain is this job of the afferents of these frameworks, being the tangible part returning to the mind. So the dorsal vagus originates from a territory that is dorsal to the core uncertain.

The Role of the Dorsal Vagal and Pain

Holding those particular subtleties is truly not significant in light of the fact that they're extremely insignificant to understanding the capacity. The capacity that we start understanding is that the core ambiguous vagal filaments are connected with the face and influence that we ordinarily have, while the dorsal vagal strands are all the more overwhelmingly connected to regions underneath the stomach. Gastric torments, touchy inside, every one of these things that are truly manifestations of different disorders that numerous individuals who endure injury has, are truly pointers of an atypical guideline of the dorsal vagus.

This turns out to be extremely significant in light of the fact that inside the model of the Polyvagal Theory, both the thoughtful sensory system and the dorsal vagus can be enlisted as protection frameworks. At the point when the ventral vagus is truly working at an elevated level and managing great, at that point, the sympathetic are simply part of the homeostatic procedures. They bolster wellbeing, development, and rebuilding. They additionally bolster development without being a protection framework.

Significance of Ventral Vagal Activity to avert Defense and Shutdown

So also a similar analogy works for the dorsal vagus. The dorsal vagus is basic; it is anything but an awful framework; however, it's not beneficial for that framework to be utilized or enlisted as a safeguard. That turns out to be extremely, the essential issue and the Polyvagal Theory gives you the various leveled model. It says, as long as the ventral vagus is truly in direction or running, at that point, your sympathetic can move any way they need in a progressively homeostatic manner to advance bloodstream and advance solid development and reclamation. It's just when the ventral vagus gets withdrawn that we get into this helplessness of a thoughtful safeguard framework. At the point when that doesn't work well, the dorsal vagus is the main thing you have left and that closes you down. You start seeing the progressive way that things work.

What is extremely significant is the job of the vagal afferents from the gut, from the sub stomach. Their job in the tweak of agony is a piece of this present part's accentuation. Diminish noticed the way that the vegas nerve, the biggest nerve in the entire human body is 80% afferent, when we see what happens when individuals stall out in the dorsal vagal framework. Steve has underlined its administrative capacity, both the dorsal vagal and the thoughtful, and obviously the ventral vagal. Yet, there are numerous circumstances, especially injury and agony

- where this guideline isn't generally homeostatic, where it's maladaptive.

Methodologies to Shift out of Maladaptive Defense States

One of the manners in which that we can change out of those maladaptive states, because of injury or pain, is through invigorating these afferents. There are a few different ways - one, for instance, is the utilization, for instance, of vibrating a sound, directly from the instinctive zone where you appear to be animating those afferents. At times you'll see an individual go from shut down and into harmony.

Thoughtful hyper excitement is an integral part of this substantial autonomic example of supporting, of choking, of holding. This prompts torment and that torment itself brings on additional propping and further actuation of the thoughtful framework. At the point when the supporting example and the torment itself have become increasingly intense, the body closes down additional into what Steve has discussed as a metabolic retreat, a condition of vitality preservation. Simultaneously, probably, that improves the arrival of endorphins, which are the body's very own narcotic agony calming framework.

Moving out of Shutdown and Working with the Sympathetic Responses Underneath

As it were, individual movements from intense agony, to intense moving towards constant, and that is the thoughtful excitement/supporting example. At that point, after some time, it goes into the shutdown. So as to help individuals, when they've been in the shutdown, we need to figure out how to help get them a tad out of the shutdown and afterward utilize the thoughtful response under that. As Steve was stating, a great deal of that guidelines originates from that ventral vagal social commitment framework, by the advisor truly being available and having the option to direct them through those excitement sensations.

Researchers concur on the significant intercession of paunch breathing or stomach relaxing. A significant number of the extremely incredible afferents identified with relaxing for the ventral vagal system are really implanted in the stomach. The issue is, we can utilize a willful framework, which means control of the stomach and breathing, or possibly deliberate breathing, to drive the stomach down and to expand the span of exhalations just as to improve or build stomach relaxing. That, as it were, expands the ventral vagal stream. Once more, the fundamental hidden subject here is that the sympathetic in the dorsal vagal framework will work in a great homeostatic manner as long as the ventral vagus is truly working. Diminish has appeared in a solid manner that you can recover a portion of this control through a deliberate breathing system.

Since what that is doing is practically setting off the ventral vagus to empower the dorsal vagus and the sympathetic to return into a homeostatic circumstance. Propping, which obviously, is an increase in engine tone, is a thoughtful assembly and that has momentary impacts, as Levine proposes, "In case I'm holding my clench hands and planning, I am fundamentally saying to my ventral vagal framework, 'Leave since I'm in a guard mode.' Now, if this doesn't dispose of the agony, since I'm in a progressive framework, or I am a various leveled framework, I've just discarded, disposed of the ventral vagus as an alternative. On the off chance that this doesn't work, what does my sensory system do? It goes down to its most minimal level."

We can't state that all the dorsal vagal reactions are negative in light of the fact that there is a level of absence of pain and now and again there is separation and no sentiment of agony. Yet, the expense of social collaboration is a cataclysmic cost to pay. When working with a customer, it's imperative to respect and regard the requirement for that specific guard framework and afterward step by step help the customer to move out of it to a less, more progressively contemporary framework, a present time and place framework.

Attention was payed to that a ton of advisors downgrade the freeze reaction and are practically phobic about it. They don't need the customer to be in a frozen state. It's critical to comprehend what sort of psycho-instruction we can give customers about how the freeze has been important to them.

Diminish includes that the freeze is a versatile reaction, implying that it has the versatile capacity and that is a piece of the psycho instructive part. At the point when individuals begin to comprehend that their body has responded, truly, in an anticipated and versatile way, it's not willful conduct. You can say: "Well mastered, I in the event that I would not like to close down; I shouldn't have closed down." But shut down is anything but an intentional framework. The body is getting things done outside the domains of mindfulness. Despite the fact that we don't know about the triggers that put us into these physiological states, the afferent input of our physiological moves positively is inside the domain of our mindfulness.

The issue is how would we name those physiological reactions? Do we reveal to ourselves that we accomplished something incorrectly or do we attempt to state, "Look, my body's accomplishing something? It might have been successful for an intense and versatile reaction, however clearly in the incessant one, the body should be corrected to state: 'Hello, it's sheltered, leave there.' Another significant factor is that when somebody leaves the shutdown, you ordinarily hear, "I didn't hurt that much previously." When the separation and the absence of pain break up, there's agony both physically and inwardly. As experts, we need to utilize instruction that fundamentally clarifies it that way. At that point, we must be available and accessible to help them at that point work through the torment. Nothing is settled - torment and injury issues don't resolve when the individual's in the shutdown - that will possibly occur on the off chance that they need to turn out enough to enable them to be vivaciously open.

Dwindle concurs that advisors are frequently awkward with the shutdown to arrange. This is likely because of a couple of variables. One is if specialists are scared of the freeze in themselves, of their own interior state. Another is that they basically don't have the foggiest idea of what to do. Most advisors are humane; they're giving it a second thought and, for the most part, well-tuned in for the customers. In the event that that is everything they do, in any case, it won't be adequate for somebody who's in a shutdown state.

The Importance of Breathing and Movement

There are various approaches to work with that, through the "voo" sound and immobilizing the jaw. For instance, the sort of breathing, that is discussed, is to utilize something like "Vooooooo." When the customer is approached to make the "voo" sound with you, you're associating the gut and afterward activating the jaw to help discharge the shutdown and freeze. Frequently in treatment, the customers are fundamentally drooped over like this. Regardless of whether the advisor says "Allows simply stroll around the room together", some of the time that is sufficient to deliver them out of their shutdown enough to begin reaching once more, it was looked at getting guidelines that should be amicable by moving among thoughtful and dorsal vagal and ventral vagal. To state it another way, we help customers to have the experience of being in the now.

Another measurement is included, which is working with facial muscles. This is a piece of what he calls the incorporated social commitment framework, which is giving enormous tangible criticism to the brain stem territory, directing the ventral vagus. It includes utilizing laryngeal, pharyngeal, trigeminal, and facial muscles in addition to tuning in. It's a coordinated framework.

Relaxing

Incredible specialist clarifies that is extremely great about breathing that we don't consider it when we do it. "We can think and do it another way, so it resembles a framework that we can actually venture into our body and change an unconstrained physiological framework. In the event that you watch customer's breath, or watch an on-edge individual, or a discouraged individual or an individual who is absolutely dissociative, you can really observe diverse breathing examples. A few scientists have really spent his life watching these kinds of things. We can look as an individual gets on edge, the breathing climbs their chest as they're truly getting shallow breaths, however, what happens is losing the chance of getting the critical impact of the stomach afferents going upwards to the ribs. All the more critically, the individual is lessening the span of the exhalation in the breath. It is during that exhalation that the ventral vagus can have a relieving impact.

At the point when analyst doing their breathing utilizing voo sounds, he is accentuating the breath out in light of the fact that else you would not have the sound; he's not sounding on the inward breath, he's sounding on the exhalation and he's empowering his customers and the advisors who utilize this system to broaden the span of their sounds. The expanded span of the exhalation implies from a polyvagal point of view, we broaden the effect of the ventral vagus."

Afferents

The contrast among afferents and Afferents by clarifying that the expression "efferent" implies that these are the nerves that are going from the mind, the brain stem for this situation, down to the viscera. "For instance, in the event that I willfully advise this hand to go into a clench hand, I'm doing that through Inference. Presently I'm shutting my eyes and I'm directing Beethoven's Fifth Symphony and afterward blast, 'If you don't mind, help me God,' I couldn't do that without afferents. Afferents are sending data from my muscles and my joints and furthermore from the viscera that educates me regarding my inward state. This can't be overstressed in sentiments of goodness and completeness – how significantly they are identified with our interior state. These receptors that are in the organs, which are in the muscles that are in the joints, are returning from the outskirts into the centrum, the mind, and the brain stem. This gives us information on who we are inside ourselves."

Some specialist includes that the afferents from the subdiaphragmatic region are once in a while perceived. "We know about it when it will, in general, be on the negative side. Subdiaphragmatically, when things are going extraordinary and the afferents and efferent are doing the suitable guideline, we're ignorant of it. Our mindfulness accompanies torment and inconvenience.

The part that I truly need to underscore is the place we have a brilliant jargon of outer sensation; we have an extremely constrained jargon for the viscera since we don't have the particularity of the instinctive receptors. It's not so much that we don't have every one of the words; we don't have all the attentive sentiments. At the point when we state 'I feel full in the wake of eating,' a portion of that isn't even an instinctive reaction. Some of it is really the stretch on the skin of our stomach area, which isn't originating from inside our guts; it's originating all things considered."

The principal year of Somatic Experiencing is finding out about those hundred, or thousands of various types of inside sensations and what they mean. We're figuring out how to explore them in the internal scene and obviously torment and injury and shut-down significantly moves you away from that procedure. It gives you this one experience of misery in the gut rather than the many subtlety sensation-based emotions that exude from a center instinctive feeling of ourselves.

Aggravation

Aggravation assumes a major job in torment. This area of our introduction thinks about how the autonomic sensory system directs agony and irritation. It begins by getting some information about the vagus nerve having receptors, some of which are influenced by cytokines, the resistant framework for incendiary action. At the point when a portion of the receptors activated by confined cytokines, discharge, this really illuminates the mind to discharge those equivalent sorts of synthetics midway. It's sort of a switchboard, so you have a receptor down beneath to get something and it sends the message "upstairs." It doesn't really go up the nerve in the feeling of the substance going up there. It's really a code.

When discussing irritation in the autonomic sensory system, the expression "ANS" might be excessively prohibitive. It was utilized the so called extended autonomic sensory system (see section 2). That term joins neuroendocrine and invulnerable and even adult individuals use as far as neuropeptides, similar to oxytocin and vasopressin. The explanation these structures are remembered for the extended ANS is that they're using comparative mind stem territories for guidelines. The apportioning of these controls, regardless of whether through psychoneural immunology or psychoendocrinology or psychophysiology demonstrate division with discrete ward factors, yet on the off chance that you take a gander at the guidelines frameworks, they're all covering.

The HPA (Hypothalamic Pituitary Adrenal Axis)

The piece of the mind that is a sort of driver of these autonomic and endocrine frameworks is the thing that has recently been known as the hypothalamic pituitary adrenal pivot (HPA). At the point when you have moved in autonomic action, you likewise get parallel moves in this hypothalamic-pituitary-adrenal hub (HPA), which influences not just irritation through the corticosteroid framework for instance, however practically the entirety of the inside metabolic and endocrinological exercises. It's extremely critical to comprehend this clinically. At the point when you work with a customer and you're working principally with their autonomic signs. At the point when they get guidelines there, all the time, individuals with immune system ailments or powerless insusceptible reactions will move. When we work with this focal pivot, a wide range of things can occur. W.R. Hess, who won the Nobel Prize in 1949, indicated that the nerve center really influences for all intents and purposes all aspects of the mind and the sensory system in the body. It is surprising that individuals don't speak much about that any longer.

Hess won the Nobel Prize in 1949 for his work on the focal guideline of the viscera. In the main passage of his discourse, he depicts how everything is interrelated to everything else in the body. He is stating that the connection among the parts is substantially more than the entirety of the little segments. Diminish and I am enormous adherents to his work.

The Dorsal Vagas and Nociception as a Cause of Pain

There's a great deal of installed look into drifting around in neurophysiology on the connection between the afferents of the dorsal vagus and nociception (the encoding and preparing of destructive boosts in the sensory system, and in this way the body's capacity to detect potential damage). Something revealed is that the tactile piece of the vagus associates with a spinal pathway that is engaged with nociception. That gets fascinating regarding develops or ideas like fibromyalgia, which will, in general, be connected particularly with individuals who have encountered significant shutdown and are truly coasting between a dorsal state and a thoughtful state. They're closing down. In the event that you just followed their colon, you'd presumably observe a similar wonder. It could be said going among obstruction and looseness of the bowels; you'd locate a similar representation at a lower level. What you need to comprehend is that two or three things get truly activated because of the changing in the afferent guideline of the autonomic sensory system while in a dorsal vagal state.

That implies that the framework that manages circulatory strain guidelines, the baroreceptors, gets disturbed. Individuals frequently get dazed and drop. They become "vasovagal thoughtful," they fall, and this is because of vagal afferents. It's a framework that isn't connected, so just a piece of it is working. Individuals regularly displaying these issues may have hypotension or hypertension. It's the circulatory strain guideline. Hess found the connection between ceaseless weakness disorder and pulse guideline issues that they are a piece of a similar system.

We may have three disorders connected together as far as symptomatology. One is the interminable weakness which will be an indication of numerous individuals who have an injury or who have encountered drawn-out periods in dorsal vagal states. The second is pulse guideline, not hypertension, yet actually getting dazed when holding up. This isn't the sort of unsteadiness where things are turning, however, where the individual truly begins hitting the ground. The third connection is fibromyalgia. These are no different systems - fibromyalgia, incessant weakness, and pulse guideline - that have gone hypotensive. This is all piece of the dorsal vagus framework, in the sense, being the final retreat and being utilized in a guarded mode.

These three troubles are aspects of a similar disorder. These side effects were deconstructed, so we can discuss every one of these indications and how they would depict fibromyalgia, circulatory strain guideline, and ceaseless exhaustion. In the event that the individual is spending a lot of their neuro-guideline time in a dorsal vagal express that isn't secured with the highlights of wellbeing, we can't immobilize unafraid.

Dread and Depression, Polyvagal Science, and Pain

Extraordinary analyst accentuates dread and wretchedness as far as polyvagal science and torment. Frequently when the torment gets interminable, the adjustment to allostatic load (the mileage on the body because of incessant pressure) is to move towards shutdown. This happens in light of the fact that there is dread related to the heap and sorrow that will, in general, fortify itself. Ordinarily, in creatures that are undermined, or under life risk won't move. They give off an impression of being dead. Much the same as a gazelle that will be brought somewhere near a cheetah. There's no development; however, then minutes after the fact, the creature just bounces up and goes off on its way. Since those states are ordinarily time-restricted. Be that as it may, when you bring dread into the stability circuit, it keeps up idleness or freeze; however, it keeps up it powerfully.

How about we take a guinea pig for a model, at the point when you take the guinea pig and grasp it, it gets stable. At that point in almost no time, seconds to minutes, it springs up and goes off. Be that as it may, on the off chance that you scare it each time it goes in, it remains longer. What could be five minutes or seven seconds, with the dread included, can for all intents and purposes keep it uncertainly. Subside did an analysis like that in Brazil and had the creature remain in that state for 24 hours. In some cases, creatures will really bite the dust. Dangers and Benefits in Coming Out of Immobility

At the point when an individual starts to leave fixed status, clinically, there's a surge of hyper excitement. Porges was discussing the thoughtful and dorsal vagal framework being in this sort of flip-flop. What you need to do is help the individual contain the thoughtful framework, by keeping them connected socially in the present time and place. At that point, there is a guideline and the stationary individual can leave the fixed status, out of the dorsal vagal shutdown, in light of the fact that they're not reactivating themselves. On the off chance that the agony turns out to be increasingly intense, you need to state: "OK".

In the event that that agony turns out to be progressively intense and you simply start to see that somewhat more, you notice if it's proceeding to increment if it's beginning to diminish or in the event that it continues as before or on the off chance that it changes to something different". With this sort of greeting, customers get the feeling that time moves along and blast, before they know it, they've left from the stability state.

It has been clarified that a few warm-blooded animals, through phylogenetic advancement, can go all through polyvagal responses as versatile capacities. Little rodents additionally do this: in any case, even in going into the dorsal vagal reaction for a little rat, there's a danger of dropping dead. The equivalent is valid with the guinea pig; there is an opportunity simply dropping dead from the immobilization reaction. This probability will, in general, happen with mice and other little rodents. What gives off an impression of being versatile can likewise be deadly; as warm-blooded creatures, we need bunches of oxygen, and when we go into shutdown states, we're not supporting our life needs just as our body needs.

Another part to recall is the thought of when the creatures leave dorsal vagal states, they shut down and they get profoundly immobilized. There is likewise a feeling of an exceptionally prepared state for some versatile reasons, and one is simply to getaway. They are attempting to recover the blood into their muscles, over into their bodies with the goal that they presently have the suitable metabolic assets to move the muscles. You have these jerks and different things that are happening as you refuel the body. At that point, the guideline begins happening. For whatever length of time that people who have recently experienced closed down are assembled, which implies that they are in a condition of frenzy or turmoil, they won't shut down. You need to consider these to be as having versatile highlights. They are not so many highlights of good social communication, yet they keep them out of closing down. Our sensory system has advanced, perfectly and articulately to move among assembly and social collaboration. That characterizes how warm-blooded creatures work and develop and endure, on the grounds that they needed to recognize quickly, who was protected and who was undependable.

The Dorsal Vagus, Goodness, and Help with Pain

Dwindle follows up prior exchange to speak all the more explicitly about the way that numerous advisors, when they find out about the dorsal vagal framework, and its focal job in injury and in ceaseless torment, will consider it to be the adversary. It's practically similar to "well, on the off chance that we could remove it, is there any valid reason why you wouldn't simply remove it?" Why not cut out those afferent and efferent associations? The explanation is that the dorsal vagal framework in vertebrates or people is extremely integral to essential sentiments of goodness and furthermore underpins sentiments of association through the ventral vagal framework. At the point when you feel warm and upbeat, you can get an aching "God; it'd be superb in the event that we could return to our strolls on the seashore, etc." Feelings of joy and those emotions, they originate from the gut. They originate from the stomach and they originate from the heart. What we're discussing is a framework that is so essential for our very own working, yet can so promptly get maladaptive and specialists need to comprehend and hold together the two sides of this.

"Wouldn't we be able to remove it? Wouldn't we be able to discourage it?" They are feeling the loss of the entire comprehension of what's happening and that is the reason if that framework is utilized as a cautious framework, it can't be a framework that supports our homeostatic needs. The equivalent is valid for the sympathetic. To conceptualize this present, a term wasn't preferred much called "Autonomic Balance." Autonomic Balance alluded to the way that as it were you have enough sympathetic and enough parasympathetic. Rather Porges stresses that "On the off chance that the ventral vagal circuit is truly working great, at that point sub diaphragmatically you have [organically] autonomic harmony between the sympathetic and the dorsal vagus."

This is the sort of equalization you need to have and this advances nice sentiments. He notes that there was an inclination of prosperity and how that climbs the afferent vagus from the gut and truly rules our capacity to get to various regions of our mind. We should not overlook this enormous progression of tangible data that is basically originating from underneath the stomach that is really changing the availability to different pieces of our brain. It's a screen.

The main problem is the capacity to keep the thoughtful and dorsal frameworks out of guarded jobs. They will be utilized for resistance at different occasions just as for their versatile capacities and on the off chance that they're intense, the parity presumably will be okay, particularly the sympathetic. On the off chance that it's drawn out, and if the sympathetic doesn't work to get us out of threat, we get into this dorsal resistance framework. That is truly where we get into issues.

Our life structures naturally close things down. In case we're not in a cautious mode, the agony isn't brought about by something natural. That all the time is the point at which you can have the individual interface with some instinctive sentiments of goodness, of alright ness of prosperity, to move to and fro between those sensations and the territory of the body where the torment is. "Ok, so you feel that torment in your shoulder, in your correct shoulder, yet then you additionally feel that sentiment of warmth and extension in your paunch. On the off chance that you let yourself move between these two sensations, notice what occurs, what changes, and afterward, what occurs straightaway?" You can enroll in those nice sentiments. Be that as it may, once more, if the body is truly in extreme agony and it gets incessant, the customer is going to be in a shutdown state.

A great many people think about whether there's a science behind this in light of the fact that there are many investigations that view the incitement of vagal afferents as mediators or modulators of physical torment. Levine is proposing that we can move our instinctive sentiments to manage the torment, how about we take an inclination that includes a subdiaphragmatic gut reaction that changes the afferent stream, changing our real state to make it simpler to manage the agony. Similarly, as though we would get the medical procedure (I'm sharing my very own arrangement of encounters here) in a confiding in the way, our tissue is extremely substantially more malleable. We won't scar to such an extent and we'll mend sooner.

The issue is trusting and feeling great, having nice sentiments. Utilizing those mental develops in explicit physiological states, distinctive tactile afferents are regulating our torment receptors and balancing the receptors of safeguard on the tissue level. We have a barrier on various levels. The body responds progressively from, it could be said, social correspondence of parts of the body, much the same as the polyvagal theory. At that point, it goes down as it ensures its components and afterward, at long last, it implodes. It goes into a real existence danger mode and implodes.

According to, Bob Naviaux, who is a doctor who runs the metabolic mitochondrial center at U.C. San Diego, microbes pursue the Polyvagal Theory. He says, "When things are great and when it's everything clear" is the representation he employs. "They converse with one another, they're intuitive. They are socially captivating." Now present a risk to the framework and it essentially makes its own protections. At that point, you can close them down, they implode and they cease to exist. The allegory of security socialization is as it were a representation of the human body at all levels.

This is a piece of the investigations of the small scale bile. This gets us back to the gut and the afferents. On the off chance that you signal that the stomach related framework will close down, creatures start dropping their pulses, and go into a shutdown response – this occurs with mice. The sign of the gut is currently passed on up the vagus to the brain stem saying: "Hello, this is awful!" Now we're examining techniques for turning around the intense injury, by essentially sending a sign up the gut saying: "Hello, everything's unmistakable." There are pharmaceutical or pharmacological strategies for sending an "all reasonable" reaction through the gut, through the receptors of the gut.

We're going to truly do an examination that applies an intense injury to the prairie vole, through limitation and predator. We essentially put him in a limitation, which is awful enough. At that point, we put his characteristic predator, a ferret, before them. A portion of their basal pulses are 400; some of them simply get tachycardia. They go up to 600. Be that as it may, others go down to 150 beats for each moment, some shutdown and seem as though they're dead. Be that as it may, there is likewise species decent variety.

It might be said, this makes the adaptively of animal types to endure. The issue of what we need to consider is at one time that vole has gone into shutdown, what befalls their social conduct, their parenting conduct? We need to invert it by sending a gut reaction up to the brain, "State, hello, your gut's everything great." Will that be adequate to turn them around?

There is a medication that animates the typical motioning of the gut that all is well, yet that is not the sole arrangement since it's a multifaceted issue as injury seems to be. He's likewise utilizing highlights of medications that he has created with acoustic incitement offering prompts to the vole in light of the fact that the voles are vocal and they vocalize as their very own sign autonomic state. On the off chance that they're worried, the prosodic element of the vole vocalization exhibits that.

Functional Ways of Shifting Out of the Freeze

Diminish has discovered that occasionally it's conceivable to do various things with activating. He has a gadget that resembles a little trampoline, yet it's totally unique. It doesn't utilize any springs and it has flexible bungee ropes. Presently when somebody remains on this, one arrives at a spot where he/she starts to, as it were, have cooperation with the trampoline. It feels like that the trampoline needs to move you a smidgen, to ricochet you a little minuscule piece and as you feel that skipping, you're getting new proprioceptive data, assembling data from the joints, from the muscles. Diminish works with individuals in serious shutdown, and accepts that doing verbal treatment could go on until the following century! Simply getting these little developments on this trampoline takes them out enough so they're available to versatility and you can work with them. It's great to recall that there are non-verbal and development situated methods for doing this.

Porges' viewpoint is consistently to deconstruct what is by all accounts attempting to give it a physiological approval. Where instincts appear to be truly on target, would we be able to give a motivation behind why? There are two things. One is shaking. Many people who have these encounters will regularly do things like this, and they need to comprehend that they are animating vagal afferents and attempting to direct circulatory strain through the development of their body in space. It's not simply body and space. They are really animating the carotid baroreceptors. It's mitigating for individuals to shake. We need to consider it to be a neural exercise, as an endeavor to restore a framework that has been down controlled.

Another way brings up the entire issue of the pelvic floor. A great deal of people who have injury encounters understands that a large number of these injury encounters will be precisely related, particularly stomach medical procedure or sub-stomach medical procedure. The pelvic floor is going to, it might be said, quit working. We need to comprehend that the pelvic floor is, as a similitude, a stomach. Similarly, as our stomach is to our lungs, the pelvic floor is to our bladder and colon.

It makes a negative weight. The pelvic floor contracts, so everybody who has had pelvic floor issues is told, "Do Kegel works out." But Kegel practices are sphincter muscles. The pelvic floor isn't a sphincter muscle, it has sphincter muscles crossing it. How would you get the pelvic floor to change and work? You do that through moving parity or parity challengers. This resembles the methodology with the trampoline. We may likewise utilize the BOSU, which is half of an activity ball.

Subside concurs that simply sitting on a gymnastic ball and making little developments, and afterward finding support to discover the sentiment of giving up the pelvic floor into the ball can truly move things. On the off chance that the individual enables the ball to help the pelvic stomach, the stomach just unwinds into the ball. You see this regularly with sexual injury, stomach medical procedures, etc.

Porges saw that Levine shut his eyes while depicting this procedure. His eyes began to hang and close.

That helped to remember the way that he had a medical procedure and I didn't care for what they instructed him to do, to manage the pelvic floor issues, so he made his very own model. He likewise understood that in the event that he shut his eyes, it was increasingly troublesome and testing, and it was working better since he was not utilizing the obvious prompts. It's ideal to work with customers with their eyes open and something to clutch. It makes a connectedness on the off chance that you are with someone else. You can even give them your arm to clutch with the goal that when they leave shut down, there you are.

Substantial Resources of the Dorsal Vagal

From Porges' perspective, it's a troublesome inquiry. It could be said, it's our center or our base of being alive and the issue is that when we attempt to utilize it as an asset, it's practically similar to utilizing it as a resistance. Rather, we need to sustain it. At the point when we support it, it serves us and this is the place the afferents are returning saying: "all unmistakable". The "every single clear" afferent are similar afferents that help our capacity to draw in others and our capacity to get to different territories of the mind that are both social and innovative. On the off chance that the sign from the dorsal vagus is, "I'm in a difficult situation," it will down direct everything else. It's an emotionally supportive network, an asset framework, whereby giving; we get, instead of a feeling of abuse from it.

The Dorsal Vagal Shutdown

The last subject for this discourse is, what counsel would you provide for specialists who are working with customers with ceaseless serious agony that gives off an impression of being identified with the dorsal vagal shutdown protective reaction? Where might you propose they start?

The dorsal-vagal shutdown reaction is looking down, looking anyplace else. You can simply tell they are going into a freeze since they are unbending and very de-centered, we as a whole realize what it resembles.

Dwindle proposes saying: "It appears as though it's extremely hard for you to talk at this moment, if that is valid, what about both of us simply stroll around the room a bit." When I lived in Colorado full time, and on the waterway, I would take customers out into the yard on the property and stroll around the stream. You could simply observe things move. Development additionally brings out interest. In any case, regardless of whether they can get inquisitive about the shutdown at that point, you've enrolled them as a partner. They watch themselves as a partner. On the off chance that somebody is in a shutdown, it's not simply freezing. It's more identified with the thoughtful despite the fact that it has segments of both.

I think the basic thing here is that when the individual is in the breakdown when you can't utilize your intelligence to get the individual to move, or inhale, and commonly when an individual has been tremendously damaged, particularly explicitly, to make a voo sound toward the start would be excessive. Strolling around the room is probably going to be alright, perhaps in any event, hopping a smidgen on that trampoline that I talked about. Once more, you can be there and hold their hand while they're doing it and afterward, when they show fervor, state "Amazing, that is awesome, appears as though you are truly feeling more vitality." You have to reach. On the off chance that its stresses they have, they need to discuss their stresses. On the off chance that its agony and what impact it has on their life, at that point let them talk about that for some time and afterward get the chance to "Alright, so now we should start to take care of that; would you say you are energetic about me?"

For whatever length of time that you make them move in a manner that isn't a battle flight development, they are going to avoid profound separation or closing down in light of the fact that, as we've stated, there's a chain of command in physiological states and on the off chance that you move you can't close down. On the off chance that you can move now in a socially strong condition, you're presently playing out a sort of neural exercise and one where the individual is picking up the capacity to move more with regards to play than they were in battle or flight.

For whatever length of time that you can remain in a moving state, without going into fight/flight, at that point, there is the chance of enrolling the social commitment frameworks and the ventral vagus since that is the gateway we have. We don't have a decent entryway of going straightforwardly out of the dorsal vagus. What we have is a gateway that in case we're gently prepared, we can push individuals or trigger individuals into increasingly social commitment.

Attention was called to that without the social vagal framework being on the web somehow or another, at any rate in connection to you as an expert, at that point the customer will most likely be unable to move out of the dorsal vagal reaction, particularly since there is no immediate entry to come legitimately out of shutdown and stability guards. The polyvagal theory advises us that the other point that is extremely basic is that when individuals are incautious states, they're going to peruse impartial signs in your face and in your conduct as negative. You must be cautious about losing contact, not being available and dismissing, doing trifling things that typically would not make any difference. Customers may, as it were, exaggerate and turn out to be exceptionally responsive and afterward vanish again on the mental level.

Dwindle makes reference to that everything is somewhat one-sided towards bogus positives. That is the reason seen danger is an endurance reaction. You generally have your discernment. I was simply expounding on this, on the memory book. Laura and I were altering this segment of the book and we took a break, strolling around. We were in Zurich, one of the most delightful of parks. We're strolling and clasping hands, and unexpectedly, we're ready to readiness. We're loathing each other's organization, No all the more clasping hands and strolling, presently, the two of us are looking and filtering – it's just as there is some frightful danger. We saw around 20 bamboo branches; the children are waving them around and not complying with the ordinary Swiss standards.

Presently recall that we feel that Zurich is the most secure spot on the planet. A recreation center like this is presumably about the most secure park in the most secure spot in the whole world. In any case, we are customized to anticipate the most noticeably terrible. We are modified to anticipate dangers. When we understood what it was, we chuckled and returned along our way. In any case, on the off chance that you've been undermined and harmed by an individual, any small seemingly insignificant detail about their face that reminds you even remotely is going to trigger them. You can't stay away from it totally, so you may, in some cases, ask, "It appears as though something I said or didn't state, appeared to disrupt the general flow, or influence you?" Again, you're helping them articulate a portion of this, which likewise is a method for bringing the frontal brain on the web and the social commitment framework on the web.

Another piece of experience is the acoustic condition. Individuals tend not to stress that. At the point when you're in a hyper-careful express, your hearing gets one-sided towards low recurrence sounds or shrill ones. It loses its keenness in the scope of prosodic highlights of a human voice. We lose incomprehension, or we hose our capacity to comprehend others' effects around us on the grounds that the low frequencies are triggers of predators. The high frequencies are triggers of somebody in torment, when those bamboo grasses, which weren't grass however 20 feet high – when they were moving, there was most likely a low recurrence murmur that was originating from them. That, to all warm-blooded animals, is predatorial. The body is modified to respond naturally to predators.

This part has exhibited a powerful discourse of the dorsal vagal segment of the polyvagal framework and its unpredictable collaborations with the ventral vagal social commitment framework and with the thoughtful/adrenal battle flight arrangement of guard and guideline.

One of the most significant rules that were underlined on numerous occasions in various manners is the significance of acquiring security through ventral vagal social commitment. In the treatment of injury and agony, this must be practiced by guiding the mending relationship through what was named "natural discourteousness" as meaningful gestures are misconstrued, acoustical sounds are seen as hazardous and predatorial, and the two individuals from the relationship are activated to pull back

Despite the fact that this is incredibly testing work, there is a lot of expectation in the procedures offered here. The endowment of basic nearness can support resistance and shutdown move to the association and recuperate. Stomach breathing and "voo" sounding expand the exhalation and the relieving sentiment of ventral vagal commitment. Basic development, like strolling around the workplace can help customers who have incredible trouble with social commitment through "eye to eye" connection and other associations. We can help thoughtful regulation by training jargon to our customers so they can remain associated with their very own body understanding and to us. Empowering development on an activity ball or extraordinary trampoline that is protected and expands social commitment is enormously mending. Delicate shaking developments can comparably be a protected and agreeable approach to enter the ventral vagal framework while starting to move out of shutdown. At last, keeping an eye on the acoustic condition and improving the prosodic characteristics of the advisor's voice can likewise extend the ventral vagal commitment, so each of the three branches helps move the living being into homeostasis and completeness.

CHAPTER NINE: CLINICAL APPLICATIONS OF THE POLYVAGAL THEORY

Creative clinicians share their encounters coordinating Polyvagal Theory into their treatment models. Clinicians who have committed their work to bring the advantages of the Polyvagal Theory to a scope of customers have met up to present Polyvagal Theory in an innovative and individual manner. Sections on a scope of points from merciful medicinal consideration to advanced restorative connections to clinician's encounters as Parents remove from the theory the amazing impact and significance of cases and sentiments of security in the clinical setting.

Also, there are sections which: expand on the guideline of wellbeing in clinical practice with kids with misuse narratives clarify the helpful outcomes of development, cadence, and move in advancing social connectedness and versatility in injury survivors clarifies how Polyvagal Theory can be utilized to understand the neurophysiological procedures in different treatments talk about dissociative procedures and medications intended to encounter real sentiments of security and trust inspect dread of flying and how utilizing positive recollections as a functioning "base up" neuropeptide procedure may successfully down-control guard shed light on the ineffectively comprehended understanding of misery Through the bits of knowledge of creative and considerate clinicians, whose treatment models are Polyvagal educated, this book gives an available method to clinicians to grasp this noteworthy theory in their very own work.

Clinicians who have committed their work to bring the advantages of the Polyvagal Theory to a scope of customers have met up to present Polyvagal Theory in an inventive and individual way. Chapters on a scope of points from humane medicinal consideration to advanced remedial connections to clinician's encounters as Parents remove from the theory the amazing impact and significance of cases and sentiments of wellbeing in the clinical setting. Additionally, there are parts which: elaborate on the standard of security in clinical practice with youngsters with misuse histories explain the therapeutic outcomes of development, cadence, and move in advancing social connectedness and strength in injury survivors explains how Polyvagal Theory can be utilized to understand the neurophysiological procedures in different therapies discuss dissociative procedures and medications intended to encounter substantial sentiments of security and trust examine dread of flying and how utilizing positive recollections as a functioning "base up" neuropeptide procedure may successfully down-control defense shed light on the ineffectively comprehended understanding of grief through the bits of knowledge of creative and big-hearted clinicians.

Adult Attachment

The Adult Attachment Interview (AAI) is both a backbone of connection look into and a groundbreaking clinical instrument. This extraordinary book gives an intensive prologue to the AAI and its utilization as a subordinate to a scope of remedial methodologies, including cognitive-conductal treatment, psychoanalytic psycho-treatment, parent-baby psycho-treatment, home visiting programs, and strong work with regards to child care and selection.

Driving specialists give definite portrayals of clinical strategies and procedures, showed with striking case material. Grounded in inquiring about, the volume features how utilizing the AAI can improve evaluation and finding, fortify the remedial partnership, and encourage objective setting, treatment arranging, and progress checking.

Reframe Your Thinking Around Autism

The Polyvagal Theory proposes chemical imbalance is an educated reaction by the body - a consequence of the kid being in a drawn-out condition of 'battle or flight' while their sensory system is as yet creating. This section clarifies the theory in basic terms and consolidates ongoing advancements in mind versatility explore (the limit of the brain to change all through life) to give Parents and experts the devices to reinforce the kid's brain-body association and reduce the social and passionate effect of chemical imbalance.

An existence without outrage is feasible - in the event that you comprehend The Anger Fallacy. Outrage is all over - behind everything from street fierceness to wrap rage, aggressive conduct at home to universal clashes. Individuals stick to their annoyance, as an apparatus of impact and a driver of vengeance. In any case, is outrage actually ever helpful? Also, would we be able to figure out how to beat it? In this engaging and momentous book, two of Australia's driving clinical therapists adopt an extreme strategy to outrage the executives, detonating the nonsensical convictions that fuel this harmful and misjudged feeling.

Through various models from mainstream society and the counseling room, and with a sizable portion of cleverness, the creators tell the best way to battle outrage by subbing sympathy and comprehension for honorable irate decisions.

CHAPTER TEN: YOGA TREATMENT AND THE POLYVAGAL THEORY

Yoga treatment is a recently developing, automatic correlative and integrative human services (CIH) practice. It is developing in its professionalization, acknowledgment & use with a showed responsibility to setting practice principles, instructive & accreditation norms, and elevating exploration to help its viability for different populaces and conditions.

In any case, heterogeneity of training, poor detailing principles, and absence of an extensively acknowledged comprehension of the neurophysiological systems associated with yoga treatment restrain the organizing of testable speculations and clinical applications.

Currently proposed structures of yoga-put together practices center with respect to the combination of base up neurophysiological and top-down neurocognitive components. What's more, it has been suggested that phenomenology and first individual moral request can give a focal point through which yoga treatment is seen as a procedure that contributes towards eudaimonic prosperity in the experience of torment, sickness or incapacity. In this article, we expand on these systems and propose a model of yoga treatment that merges with Polyvagal Theory (PVT).

PVT joins the development of the autonomic sensory system to the rise of prosocial practices and sets that the neural stages supporting social conduct are engaged with looking after wellbeing, development and reclamation. This logical model, which associates neurophysiological examples of autonomic guidelines and articulation of enthusiastic and social conduct, is progressively used as a system for understanding human conduct, stress and disease.

In particular, we portray how PVT can be conceptualized as a neurophysiological partner to the yogic ideal of the gunas, or characteristics of nature. Like the neural stages portrayed in PVT, the gunas give the establishment from which conduct, passionate and physical traits rise. We depict how these two distinct yet closely resembling structures - one situated in neurophysiology and the other in an old intelligence convention - feature yoga treatment's advancement of physical, mental and social prosperity for self-guideline and strength. This parallel between the neural foundation of PVT and the gunas of yoga is instrumental in making a translational structure for yoga treatment to line up with its philosophical establishments. Thusly, yoga treatment can work as a particular practice instead of fitting into an outside model for its usage in inquires about and clinical settings.

Mind-body treatments, including yoga treatment, are proposed to profit wellbeing and prosperity through reconciliation of top-down and base up forms encouraging bidirectional correspondence between the brain and body. Top-down procedures, for example, the guideline of consideration and setting of expectation, have been appeared to diminish mental worry just as the hypothalamic-pituitary pivot (HPA) and thoughtful sensory system (SNS) movement, and thusly balance insusceptible capacity and irritation.

Base up forms, advanced by breathing procedures and development rehearses, have been appeared to impact the musculoskeletal, cardiovascular and sensory system work and furthermore influence HPA and SNS movement with attending changes in resistant capacity and passionate prosperity.

The top-down and base up forms utilized at the top of the priority list body treatments may control autonomic, neuroendocrine, enthusiastic and conduct actuation and bolster a person's reaction to challenges. Self-guideline, a cognizant capacity to keep up the security of the framework by overseeing or modifying reactions to risk or misfortune, may diminish side effects of differing conditions, for example, peevish inside disorder, neurodegenerative conditions, interminable agony, wretchedness and PTSD through the moderation of allostatic load with a going with the move-in autonomic state have proposed such a model of top-down and base up self-administrative components of yoga for mental wellbeing.

Versatility may give another advantage of mind-body treatments as it incorporates the capacity of a person to "ricochet back" and adjust in light of affliction as well as unpleasant conditions in an opportune manner to such an extent that psychophysiological assets are rationed. High strength is related to faster cardiovascular recuperation following abstract passionate encounters, less saw pressure, more noteworthy recuperation from ailment or injury and better administration of dementia and incessant agony. Traded off versatility is connected to dysregulation of the autonomic sensory system through proportions of vagal guidelines (respiratory sinus arrhythmia. Yoga is related to both improvement in proportions of mental strength and improved vagal guidelines.

This article investigates the mix of top-down and base up forms for self-guideline and versatility through both Polyvagal Theory and yoga treatment. PVT will be portrayed in connection to contemporary understandings of interoception just as the bioconductal theory of the "preliminary set", which will be characterized later. This will help to spread out an incorporated framework from which mind-body treatments encourage the development of physiological, enthusiastic and social qualities for the advancement of self-guideline and strength.

We will look at the union of the neural stages, depicted in PVT, with the three Gunas, a fundamental idea of yogic way of thinking that portrays the characteristics of material nature. Both PVT and yoga give structures to seeing how basic neural stages (PVT) and gunas (yoga) interface the development and availability between physiological, mental and conduct characteristics. By influencing the neural stage, or guna transcendence, just as one's relationship to the ceaseless moving of these neural stages, or gunas, the individual learns aptitudes for self-guideline and strength. In addition, these structures share qualities that parallel each other where the neural stage mirrors the guna power and the guna prevalence mirrors the neural stage.

PVT, and other rising hypotheses, for example, neurovisceral combination, help explain associations between the frameworks of the body, the brain, and the procedures of the mind offering expanded understanding into complex examples of incorporated top-down and base up forms that are natural to mind-body treatments. PVT portrays three particular neural stages in light of apparent hazard (i.e., wellbeing, peril, and life-risk) in the condition that works in a phylogenetically decided chain of command steady with the Jacksonian guideline of disintegration. PVT acquaints the idea of neuroception with depicting the subliminal recognition of wellbeing or peril in nature through base up forms including vagal afferents, tangible info identified with outside difficulties, and endocrine components that recognize and assess ecological hazard before the cognizant elaboration by higher mind focuses.

The three polyvagal neural stages, as portrayed underneath, are connected to the practices of social correspondence, guarded procedure of activation and protective immobilization:

The ventral vagal complex (VVC) gives the neural structures that intervene in the "social commitment framework". At the point when wellbeing is recognized in the interior and outside condition, the VVC gives a neural stage to help prosocial conduct and social association by connecting the neural guideline of instinctive states supporting homeostasis and reclamation to facial expressivity and the open and expressive areas of correspondence (e.g., prosodic vocalizations and upgraded capacity to tune in to voice). The engine segment of the VVC, which starts in the core ambiguous (NA) manages and organizes the muscles of the face and head with the bronchi and heart. These associations help arrange the individual towards human association and commitment in prosocial connections and give increasingly adaptable and versatile reactions to ecological difficulties including social communications

The SNS is oftentimes connected with battle/flight practices. Battle/flight practices require initiation of the SNS and are the underlying and essential guard procedures enlisted by warm-blooded creatures. This safeguard technique requires expanded metabolic yield to help activation practices. Inside PVT, the enlistment of SNS in guard pursues the Jacksonian guideline of disintegration and mirrors the versatile responses of a phylogenetically requested reaction progressively in which the VVC has neglected to alleviate risk. At the point when the SNS circuit is selected, there are monstrous physiological changes remembering an expansion for muscle tone, shunting of blood from the fringe, restraint of gastrointestinal capacity, an enlargement of the bronchi, increments in pulse and respiratory rate, and arrival of catecholamines.

This assembly of physiological assets makes way for reacting to genuine or accepted peril in the earth and towards the ultimate objectives of security and endurance. At the point when the SNS turns into the predominant neural stage, the VVC impact might be repressed for activating assets for a quick activity. Though prosocial practices and social associations are related to the VVC, the SNS is related to practices and feelings, for example, dread or outrage that help to arrange to the earth for security or wellbeing.

The dorsal vagal complex (DVC) emerges from the dorsal core of the vagus (DNX) and gives the essential vagal engine filaments to organs situated beneath the stomach. This circuit is intended to adaptably react to massive peril or dread and is the crudest (i.e., developmentally most established) reaction to stretch. Initiation of the DVC in resistance brings about an uninvolved reaction portrayed by diminished muscle tone, and emotional decrease of heart yield to save metabolic assets, modification in gut and bladder work by means of reflexive poop and pee to lessen metabolic requests required by processing.

PVT sets that through these neural stages, specific physiological states, mental traits, and social procedures are associated, develop, and are made open to the person. The physiological state built up by these neural stages in light of risk or security (as decided through the coordinated procedures of neuroception) takes into consideration or limits the scope of passionate and social attributes that are open to the person

A center part of PVT is those examples of physiological state, feeling and conduct are specific to each neural stage (for a point by point audit of the neurophysiological, neuroanatomical, and developmental natural bases of PVT. For instance, the neural foundation of the VVC is proposed to associate instinctive homeostasis with passionate qualities and prosocial practices that are contradictory with the neurophysiological states, enthusiastic attributes or social practices that show in the neural foundation of protective procedures found in SNS or DVC initiation. At the point when the VVC is predominant, the vagal brake is executed and pro-social practices and enthusiastic states, for example, association and love can possibly develop.

At the point when the SNS is the essential guarded system, the NA kills the inhibitory activity of the ventral vagal pathway to the heart to empower thoughtful enactment and social and passionate procedures of assembly are bolstered. On the off chance that the DVC idleness reaction is the cautious system, the dorsal engine core is initiated as a defensive component from agony or potential demise and dynamic reaction methodologies are not accessible.

It is imperative to take note of the VVC has different qualities that empower mixed states with the SNS (e.g., play) or with the DVC (e.g., closeness). Be that as it may, in these instances of mixed states, the VVC remains effectively available and practically contains the subordinate circuits. At the point when the VVC is practically pulled back, it advances the availability of the SNS as a guard battle/flight framework. So also, the SNS practically restrains access to the DVC immobilization shutdown reaction. In this way, the significant shutdown response that may prompt demise turns out to be neurophysiologically available just when the SNS is reflexively repressed.

Vagal Activity, Interoception, Regulation, and Resilience

Vagal movement, by means of ventral vagal pathways, is recommended to be intelligent of guideline and versatility of the framework where high heart vagal tone associated with increasingly versatile top-down and base up procedures, for example, consideration guideline, full of feeling preparing and adaptability of physiological frameworks to adjust and react to the earth. Vagal control has additionally been appeared to relate with differential actuation in mind locales that manage reactions to risk evaluation, interoception, feeling guideline, and the advancement of more noteworthy adaptability in light of challenge. On the other hand, the low vagal guideline has been related with maladaptive base up and top-down handling bringing about poor self-guideline, less social adaptability, discouragement, summed up uneasiness issue, and antagonistic wellbeing results remembering expanded mortality for conditions, for example, lupus, rheumatoid joint pain, and injury.

The vagus nerve is involved 80% afferent filaments and fills in as a significant conductor for interoceptive correspondence about the condition of the viscera and inside milieu to brain structures. Interoception has been investigated as basic to the connecting of top-down and base up preparing and in the examination of the connections between sensations, feelings, sentiments and sympathovagal. Backing has been found for the joining of interoceptive info, feeling and a guideline of sympathovagal balance in the separate and cingulate cortices, encouraging a bound together reaction of the person to body, mind or natural (BME) wonders.

Self-guideline is proposed to be subject to the precision with which we decipher and react to interoceptive data, with more prominent exactness prompting upgraded versatility and self-guideline. Thusly, interoception is viewed as significant in torment, habit, enthusiastic guideline, and solid versatile practices, including social commitment. Furthermore, interoception has been proposed as key to versatility as the precise preparation of interior substantial states advances a brisk rebuilding of homeostatic parity.

It has been suggested that mind-body treatments are a successful device for the guideline of vagal capacity, with resulting encouraging of versatile capacities including the alleviation of unfavorable impacts related with social difficulty, the decrease of allostatic load, and the assistance of self-administrative abilities and strength of the ANS crosswise over different patient populaces and conditions.

Polyvagal Theory & Mind-Body Therapies for Regulation & Resilience

Mind-body treatments underscore the development of physical mindfulness, including both interoception and proprioception, joined with the care based characteristics of non-judgment, non-reactivity, interest, or acknowledgment so as to take part in a procedure of re-evaluation of improvements. While being urged to develop familiarity with BME wonders and boosts, the individual is bolstered in a procedure of re-elucidation or re-direction to such improvements, so understanding may happen and flexibility, guideline, and versatility might be cultivated.

This ability to change the relationship and response to BME wonders is believed to be fundamental for self-guideline and prosperity. It has been indicated that patients using mind-body treatments for recuperating revealed both a move as far as they can tell and reaction to negative feelings and sensations just as the improvement of self-administrative aptitudes in managing torment, enthusiastic guideline and re-examination of life circumstances.

PVT offers knowledge into how figuring out how to perceive and move the hidden neural foundation of any given psychophysiological state may legitimately influence physiology, feeling and conduct along these lines helping the individual develop versatile procedures for guideline and flexibility to profit physical, mental and social wellbeing. As mind-body treatments influence the vagal pathways they are proposed to shape methods for "working out" these neural stages to encourage self-guideline and strength of physiological capacity, feeling guideline and prosocial practices.

Ideal neural guideline of the autonomic sensory system and the related endocrine and invulnerable frameworks is encouraged through the dynamic commitment of the VVC by using explicit developments or positions, breathing works on, reciting or contemplation which influences both top-down and base up forms.

Versatility is proposed to be cultivated by both downregulating cautious states and supporting greater adaptability and flexibility in relation to different wonders of the BME to advance physiological rebuilding just as positive mental and social states. The individual can figure out how to improve the actuation of the VVC with its homeostatic effect on the living being, just as increment the office to move all through other neural stages, for example, the SNS or DVC when genuine or saw pressure is experienced.

In total, personality body practices can show the person to make the VVC increasingly open, extend the limit of resilience to other neural stages, change the relationship and reaction to SNS and DVC neural stages that happen as common vacillations of the BME, and how to turn out to be progressively talented at moving all through these neural stages. Breathing moves inside yoga regularly encourage comparable moves in the autonomic state with focalized mental and wellbeing outcomes. These practices may likewise add to our capability to encounter association past social communications or systems and to a progressively all-inclusive and unbounded feeling of unity and association.

SUMMARY

Polyvagal Theory will control you bit by bit through four modules of top to bottom preparing to help you adequately incorporate the transformative intensity of this method and the Social Engagement System in your training. This is what's canvassed in every module:

The Polyvagal Theory

- Principles and highlights of the Polyvagal Theory, and how to apply it in a clinical setting
- How the Polyvagal Theory can demystify a few highlights identified with pressure-related sicknesses and mental issue, for example, PTSD, chemical imbalance, melancholy, and uneasiness
- How the Social Engagement System is undermined by pressure and injury and how to reset it

- Evolutionary changes and versatile capacities in the autonomic sensory system
- Humans' reaction chain of importance to challenges
- Three neural stages that give the neurophysiological bases to social commitment, battle/flight, and shutdown practices

Social Engagement System and Psychiatric and Conductal Disorders

- The "face-heart" association that structures a useful social commitment framework
- How our outward appearances, vocalizations, and signals are controlled by neural components that are engaged with managing our autonomic sensory system

Perception: Detecting and Evaluating Risk

- How our social and physical condition triggers changes in physiological state

- Understanding how versatile physiological responses may bring about maladaptive practices
- Immobilization unafraid
- Play as a neural exercise and tuning in as a neural exercise
- Fight/flight and immobilization guard methodologies
- The adaptive function of immobilization and the related clinical troubles
- How the burdens and difficulties of life mutilate social mindfulness and dislodge unconstrained social commitment practices with protective responses

Applying the Polyvagal Theory in Clinical Settings

- Understanding sound-related hypersensitivities
- State guideline as a central element of mental issue
- Deconstructing highlights of chemical imbalance and PTSD

- Strategies to clarify disturbance and fix of advantageous guideline
- Identifying expressive gestures that upset or fix cautious response

Convergence of Polyvagal Theory with the *Gunas*

Both PVT and the gunas give a point of view to comprehend fundamental establishments from which physical, mental and social traits rise. PVT gives an understanding into how hidden neural stages are enacted because of saw risk or security within sight of BME marvels. Yoga recommends that physical, mental and conduct properties rise up out of and are affected by the fundamental exchange of the gunas.

The two structures examine the conjunction and mixing together of neural stages (PVT) or gunas (Yoga) and endeavor to pass on multifaceted nature in the midst of a characteristic inclination for reductionism inside customary scholarly trains. In PVT, the conjunction of neural stages offers a route to the fluctuated encounters of play (safe preparation) and closeness (safe immobilization).

In yoga, the conjunction of the gunas makes the changed marvels of BME and impacts the relationship and response to such boosts. The two speculations encourage that it is from the surfacing of the neural foundation of PVT or the guna of yoga that BME states are made the show and set up.

The gunas of yoga and neural foundation of PVT are additionally reflected in each other in a merged and closely resembling way. This connection between the two models can be seen through the practically identical depictions of properties. At the point when the ANS goes under the impact of one of the gunas a particular neural foundation of the PVT might be initiated supporting shared qualities between the two. In like manner, when a neural stage is actuated, it bolsters the transcendence of a guna and the common attributes between them rise. For instance, when sattva reflects through the sensory system, the physiological, mental, and conduct qualities of the VVC show, or when the VVC is actuated the characteristics of sattva show, as will be depicted in more detail beneath.

This exchange investigates the connection between the two models by the way they relate and influence each other for the rise of physical, mental, and social traits. Eventually, this relationship is intended to encourage an understanding that yoga treatment may influence both basic neural stages and gunas, bringing about developed self-guideline and strength for the prosperity of the person.

Poly Faces of Vagus

There are two diverse vagus circuits - a sum of three ANS circuits, not only a couple. The two circuits "originate from two distinct regions of the brain stem, and they advanced successively," one far prior. This spurred me to build up the polyvagal theory, which revealed the life structures and capacity of two vagal frameworks, one conceivably deadly, and the other defensive.

"Immobilization, bradycardia, and apnea are segments of an old, reptilian protection framework,"

Porges says. "In the event that you take a gander at reptiles, you don't see a lot of conduct - on the grounds that immobilization is the essential barrier framework for reptiles… it's an old vagus nerve." This pre-notable nerve has no myelin, a nerve covering of defensive protein and fat.

Vertebrates have this unmyelinated vagus, on the dorsal (top) side of the nerve, which immobilizes us, as well "and that immobilization response, versatile for reptiles, is conceivably deadly for warm-blooded creatures.

It was observed that among the "firsts," which started with well-evolved creatures, another vagus with myelin creates on the ventral underside of the nerve. "So warm-blooded creatures have two vagal circuits," he found. "The myelinated circuits give progressively fast and firmly composed reactions. The new mammalian vagus is connected to brain stem zones that direct the muscles of the face and head. Each natural clinician realizes that in the event that they see individuals' appearances and tune in to voices, constrained by muscles of the face and head, they know the physiological condition of their customer."

Neuroception: It's Just Not Cognitive

Our progressively crude neural circuits work by "neuroception" - absolutely automatically. "Neuroception isn't discernment," he says. "Neuroception doesn't require consciousness of things going on. It is discovery without mindfulness. It is a neural circuit that assesses chance in the earth… When gone up against in specific circumstances, a few people experience autonomic reactions, for example, an expansion in pulse and perspiring hands. These reactions are automatic. It doesn't care for they need to do this."

The polyvagal theory stresses that our sensory system has more than one safeguard procedure - and whether we use prepared flight/flight or immobilization shutdown, is certifiably not an intentional choice. Outside the domain of our cognizant mindfulness, our sensory system is constantly assessing danger in the earth, making decisions, and organizing practices that are not subjective.

Next, he says, "people and different well evolved creatures, as battle/flight machines, possibly work in the event that they can move and get things done. Yet, on the off chance that we are restricted, in the event that we are set into confinement, or on the off chance that we are lashed down, our sensory system peruses those signs and practically needs to immobilize.

CONCLUSION

In conclusion, the polyvagal theory proposes that the evolution of the mammalian autonomic sensory system gives the neurophysiological substrates to versatile conduct procedures. It further suggests that the physiological state confines the scope of conduct and mental experience. The theory connects the advancement of the autonomic sensory system to full of feeling experience, passionate demeanor, facial signals, vocal correspondence, and unforeseen social conduct. Right now, the theory gives a conceivable clarification to the announced covariation between atypical autonomic guidelines (e.g., decreased vagal and expanded thoughtful impacts to the heart) and mental and conduct issues that include challenges in directing proper social, passionate, and correspondence practices.

The polyvagal theory gives a few experiences into the versatile idea of a physiological state. In the first place, the theory stresses that physiological states bolster various classes of conduct. For instance, a physiological state described by a vagal withdrawal would bolster the preparation practices of battle and flight. Interestingly, a physiological state portrayed by expanded vagal effect on the heart (by means of myelinated vagal pathways starting in the core ambiguous) would support unconstrained social commitment practices. Second, the theory accentuates the arrangement of a coordinated social commitment framework through useful and auxiliary connections between neural control of the striated muscles of the face and the smooth muscles of the viscera. Third, the polyvagal theory proposes an instrument – neuroception - to trigger or to restrain safeguard methodologies.